FITNESS
and
WELLNESS

SECOND EDITION

Werner W. K. Hoeger
Boise State University

Sharon A. Hoeger

D1297878

Morton Publishing Company

925 W. Kenyon Ave., Unit 12
Englewood, Colorado 80110

In memory of my father.
This was his favorite book.

With kind gratitude to the following individuals who helped make this work possible: Dan Barber, Dr. Sherman Button, Cherianne Calkins, Debra Cunningham, Neil Edwards, Jim Moore, Sally O'Donnell, Brad Page, Phyllis Sawyer, Brad Thompson, Scott Whiles, Julie Wagner, and Julie Wolf.

Printed in the United States of America

10 9 8 7 6 5 4 3 2 1

ISBN: 0-89582-256-3

Preface

More than ever before Americans realize that good health is largely self-controlled and that premature illness and mortality can be prevented through adequate fitness and positive lifestyle habits. The current American way of life, unfortunately, does not provide the human body with sufficient physical activity to maintain adequate health. Furthermore, many present lifestyle patterns are such a serious threat to our health that they actually increase the deterioration rate of the human body and often lead to premature illness and mortality.

Several major scientific research studies indicate that people who lead an active and healthy lifestyle live longer and enjoy a better quality of life. As a result, the importance of sound fitness and wellness programs has taken an entire new dimension. From an initial fitness fad in the early 1970s, healthy lifestyle programs have become a trend that is now very much a part of the American way of life.

Nevertheless, while people in the United States are firm believers in the benefits of exercise and positive lifestyle habits as a means to promote better health, most do not reap these benefits because they do not know how to implement a sound fitness and wellness program that will yield the desired results. Therefore, the information presented in this book has been written with this purpose in mind: to provide you with the necessary guidelines to implement a lifetime exercise and healthy lifestyle program so you can make a constant and deliberate effort to stay healthy and realize your highest potential for well-being.

NEW AND ENHANCED FEATURES
OF THE SECOND EDITION

The contents of this second edition of Fitness and Wellness have been revised and updated to include new and relevant information presented at professional meetings and reported in the literature over the last few years. The most significant changes of this third edition are:

■ Inclusion of the latest information available on the association between fitness and all-cause mortality and the effects of a healthy lifestyle on quality of life and longevity.

■ An introduction to physical fitness versus health fitness, including performance standards for both fitness classifications. This new addition will allow individuals to select realistic goals based on their personal philosophy of life and fitness.

■ A 1.0-mile walk test for cardiovascular endurance assessment has been added to the Chapter 2. This test is useful for individuals, who, because of physical limitations are unable to perform the 1.5-mile run test.

■ A Waist-to-Hip Ratio test developed by a panel of scientists appointed by the National Academy of Sciences and the Dietary Guidelines Advisory Council for the U.S. Departments of Agriculture and Health and Human Services has also been added to Chapter 2. This test is used to screen individuals who might be at higher risk for disease due to high abdominal fat content.

■ The cardiovascular endurance and muscular strength exercise prescriptions have been revised to conform with "The Recommended Quantity and Quality of Exercise for Developing and Maintaining Cardio-respiratory and Muscular Fitness in Healthy Adults" by the American College of Sports Medicine (ACSM).

■ A new *Exercise Readiness* questionnaire has been included in Chapter 3. This questionnaire evaluates the students' readiness for exercise based on four categories of evaluation: mastery (self-control), attitude, health, and commitment.

■ A new chapter on aerobic activity choices (Chapter 4) has been added to the book. This introduction to the most popular forms of aerobic activities will enhance the development and implementation of cardiovascular fitness programs.

■ Several additions have been made to the nutrition and weight control chapter. Information on the antioxidant role of selected vitamins and minerals, an update on the RDA (1989 version), the new Food Guide Pyramid, and an expanded list of the nutritive value of selected foods (contained in Appendix E) have been included. The ever increasing role of exercise in weight management, both aerobic and strength training, has been expanded to incorporate recent research findings in this area.

■ Major revisions have been made to the healthy lifestyle chapter (Chapter 6). Updates include data on the even stronger than previously thought relationship between HDL-cholesterol and coronary heart disease, the general recommendations by the National Cholesterol Education Program (NCEP), blood- lipid standards, antioxidant effects of vitamins and minerals, the effects of low fat diets on cholesterol levels, and the minimum exercise dose for moderate cardiovascular fitness.

■ A glossary that includes all key terms used in the text has been added at the end of the book.

■ New color photography and many outstanding new graphs have been added to the book.

SUPPLEMENTS

The following ancillaries are provided free of charge to all qualified adopters:

■ **A comprehensive computer software package** that includes a fitness and wellness profile, a personalized cardiovascular exercise prescription, a nutrient analysis, and a weekly and monthly exercise log. The fitness and wellness profile provides a pre- and post-test fitness comparison, including percent change for each fitness item on the profile.

■ A fitness assessment **video** containing a detailed explanation of the fitness tests in the book. Instructors can use this video to help familiarize themselves with the proper test protocols for each fitness test. This audio-visual aid contains the following test items: 1.5-mile run test, muscular endurance test, modified sit-and-reach test, body rotation test, and skin-fold thickness test.

■ The Morton Test II Fitness & Wellness **Computerized Testbank** with the following options: (a) over 600 multiple choice questions, (b) additional multiple choice, true-false or essay test questions can be added by the course instructors, (c) previously generated tests can be recalled — creating new exam versions since all multiple choice answers rotate with each new test generated, (d) capability to generate tests using a LaserJet printer, and (e) answer sheets can be formatted to be read by a scanner.

■ Sixty color **overhead transparency acetates** to facilitate class instruction and help explain key fitness and wellness concepts.

■ An **instructor's manual** to aid with the implementation of your fitness and wellness course.

Contents

The Importance of Physical Fitness

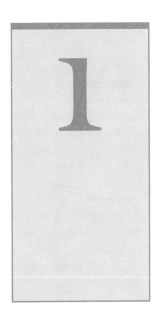

OBJECTIVES

- Understand the importance of physical fitness.
- Define physical fitness.
- Understand the wellness concept.
- Learn the benefits of a total fitness program and wellness program.
- Determine whether medical clearance is required for safe exercise participation.

During the last 25 years the number of people participating in physical fitness programs has increased tremendously. From an initial fitness fad in the early 1970s, fitness programs became a trend that is now very much a part of the American way of life. The increase in the number of fitness participants is attributed primarily to scientific evidence linking vigorous exercise and positive lifestyle habits to better health and improved quality of life.

Unfortunately, the current American way of life does not provide the human body with sufficient physical exercise to maintain adequate health. Furthermore, many lifestyle patterns are such a serious threat to our health that they actually increase the deterioration of the human body and often lead to premature illness and mortality.

Although people in the United States firmly believe in the benefits of physical activity and positive lifestyle habits as a means to promote better health, most do not reap these benefits because they do not know how to implement a sound fitness program that will yield the desired results. According to the U.S. Department of Health and Human Services, *less than half of the adult population in the United States exercises regularly and only 10 to 20% exercises vigorously enough to develop the cardiovascular system.*

Patty Neavill is a typical example of someone who frequently tried to change her life around but was unable to do so because she did not know how to implement a sound exercise and weight control program. At age 24, Patty, a college sophomore, was discouraged with her weight, level of fitness, self-image, and quality of life in general. She had struggled with weight most of her life. Like thousands of other people, she had made many unsuccessful attempts to lose weight. Patty put her fears aside and decided to enroll in a fitness course. As part of the course requirement, she took a battery of fitness tests at the beginning of the semester. Patty's cardiovascular fitness and strength ratings were poor, her flexibility classification was average, she weighed more than 200 pounds, and her percent body fat was 41.

Following the initial fitness assessment, Patty met with her course instructor, who prescribed an exercise and nutrition program like the one in this book. Patty fully committed to carry out the prescription. She walked or jogged five times a week, worked out with weights twice a week, and played volleyball or basketball two to four times each week. Her daily caloric intake was set in the range of 1,500 to 1,700 calories. She took care to meet the minimum required servings from the basic food groups each day, which contributed about 1,200 calories to her diet. The remainder of the calories came primarily from complex carbohydrates. At the end of the 16-week semester, Patty's cardiovascular fitness, strength, and flexibility ratings had all improved to the good category, she lost 50 pounds, and her percent body fat had dropped to 22.5!

A thank you note from Patty to the course instructor at the end of the semester read:

> *Thank you for making me a new person. I truly appreciate the time you spent with me. Without your kindness and motivation, I would have never made it. It is great to be fit and trim. I've never had this feeling before and I wish everyone could feel like this once in their life.*
>
> *Thank you,*
>
> *Your trim Patty!*

Patty had never been taught the principles governing a sound weight loss program. Not only did she need this knowledge, but, like most Americans who have never experienced the process of becoming physically fit, she needed to be in a structured exercise setting to truly feel the joy of fitness.

Of even greater significance, Patty has maintained her aerobic and strength-training programs. A year after ending her calorie-restricted diet, her weight increased by 10 pounds, but her body fat decreased from 22.5 to 21.2%. As discussed in Chapter 5, the weight increase is related mostly to changes in lean tissue, lost during the weight-reduction phase. Despite only a slight drop in weight during the second year following the calorie-restricted diet, the 2-year follow-up revealed a further decrease in body fat, to 19.5%. Patty understands the new quality of life reaped through a sound fitness program.

LIFESTYLE, HEALTH, AND QUALITY OF LIFE

Many research findings have shown that *physical inactivity and negative lifestyle habits are a serious threat to health.* Movement and physical activity are basic functions for which the human organism was created. Now, however, advances in modern technology have almost completely eliminated the need for physical activity in almost everyone's daily life.

Physical activity is no longer a natural part of our existence. Today we live in an automated society. Most of the activities that used to require strenuous physical exertion can be accomplished by machines with the simple pull of a handle or push of a button. For instance, if people need to go to a store that is only a couple of blocks away, most drive their automobiles and then spend a couple of minutes driving around the parking lot to find a spot 10 yards closer to the store's entrance (Figure 1.1). The groceries do not even have to be carried out any more. They usually are taken out in a cart and placed in the vehicle by a youngster working at the store.

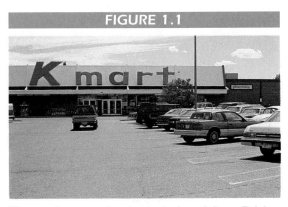

FIGURE 1.1

The epitome of physical inactivity: Driving around a parking lot for several minutes in search of a parking spot 10 to 20 yards closer to the store's entrance.

Similarly, during a visit to a multi-level shopping mall, almost everyone chooses to ride the escalators instead of taking the stairs. Automobiles, elevators, escalators, telephones, intercoms, remote controls, electric garage door openers — all are modern-day commodities that minimize the amount of movement and effort required of the human body.

One of the most significant detrimental effects of modern-day technology has been an increase in chronic conditions related to a lack of physical activity. These include hypertension, heart disease, chronic low back pain, and obesity, among others. They sometimes are referred to as hypokinetic diseases. The term "hypo" means low or little, and "kinetic" implies motion. Lack of adequate physical activity is a fact of modern life that most people can no longer avoid, but to enjoy contemporary commodities and still expect to live life to its fullest, a personalized lifetime exercise program must become a part of daily living.

With the new developments in technology, three additional factors have changed our lives significantly and have had a negative effect on human health: nutrition, stress, and environment. Fatty foods, sweets, alcohol, tobacco, excessive stress, and environmental hazards, such as wastes, noise, and air pollution, have detrimental effects on people.

As the incidence of chronic diseases increased, it became obvious that prevention was the best medicine. According to research, *more than 50% of all disease is self-controlled,* 64% of the factors contributing to mortality are caused by lifestyle (48%) and environmental (16%) factors, and *83% of deaths prior to age 65 are preventable.* Most Americans are threatened by the very lives they lead today.

The leading causes of death in the United States today are lifestyle-related (see Figure 1.2). Approximately 70% of all deaths in this country are caused by cardiovascular disease

FIGURE 1.2

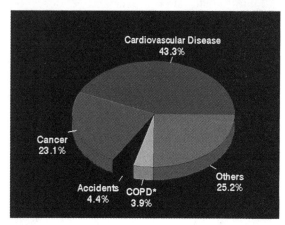

Leading causes of death in the United States: 1989.

Source: Advance Report of Final Mortality Statistics, 1989, National Center for Health Statistics, U.S. Department of Health and Human Services.

(encompassing heart disease and cerebrovascular diseases) and cancer. Nearly 80% of these deaths could be prevented through a healthy lifestyle program. Accidents are the third leading cause of death. Although not all accidents are preventable, many are. Fatal accidents frequently are related to abusing drugs and not using seat belts. The fourth cause of death, chronic and obstructive pulmonary disease, is largely related to tobacco use.

PHYSICAL FITNESS

The American Medical Association defines physical fitness as the *general capacity to adapt and respond favorably to physical effort.* This implies that individuals are physically fit when they can meet both the ordinary and the unusual demands of daily life safely and effectively without being overly fatigued, and still have energy left for leisure and recreational activities. Physical fitness can be classified into health-related and motor-skill-related fitness. From a health point of view, fitness has four health-related components (see Figure 1.3):

- *Cardiovascular endurance:* the ability of the heart, lungs, and blood vessels to supply oxygen to the cells to meet the demands of prolonged physical activity (aerobic exercise).
- *Muscular strength and endurance:* the ability of the muscles to generate force.
- *Muscular flexibility:* the capacity of a joint to move freely through a full range of motion.
- *Body composition:* the amount of lean body mass and adipose tissue (fat mass) in the human body.

FIGURE 1.3

Health-Related

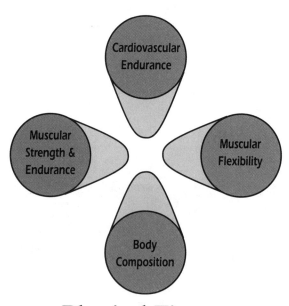

Physical Fitness

Health-related components of physical fitness.

To improve overall fitness, an individual has to participate in specific programs to develop each one of the four basic components. Nevertheless, after the initial fitness boom swept across the country in the 1970s, it became clear that improving the four components of physical fitness alone would not always decrease the risk for disease and ensure better health. As a result, a new concept developed in the 1980s that goes beyond the basic components of fitness. This concept is called *wellness*, defined as *the constant and deliberate effort to stay healthy and achieve the highest potential for well-being*.

Wellness implies an all-inclusive umbrella covering a variety of activities to help individuals recognize detrimental components of their lifestyle and implement positive behaviors that will improve health, quality of life, and total well-being. Wellness goes way beyond absence of disease and optimal fitness. It incorporates elements such as adequate fitness, proper nutrition, stress management, disease prevention, spirituality, smoking cessation, personal safety, substance abuse control, regular physical examinations, health education, and environmental support. Additional information on wellness and how to implement a wellness program is discussed in Chapter 6.

The motor skill-related components of fitness are more important in athletics than in typical living. In addition to the four components just mentioned, motor skill-related fitness includes agility, balance, coordination, power, reaction time, and speed (see Figure 1.4). Although these components are important in achieving success in athletics, they are not crucial for developing better health. In terms of preventive medicine, the main emphasis of fitness programs should be placed on the health-related components. That is the focus of this book.

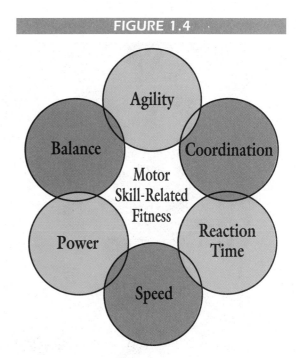

FIGURE 1.4

Motor-skill components of physical fitness.

Benefits of Fitness and Wellness

Although the benefits to be enjoyed from participating in a regular fitness and wellness program are many and indications are that active people live a longer life (see Figures 1.5 and 1.6), the greatest benefit of all is that *physically fit individuals enjoy a better quality of life*. Fit people who lead a positive lifestyle live a better and healthier life. These people live life to its fullest potential and have fewer health problems than inactive individuals who also may indulge in negative lifestyle patterns.

Although compiling an all-inclusive list of the benefits reaped through participation in a fitness and wellness program is difficult,

FIGURE 1.5

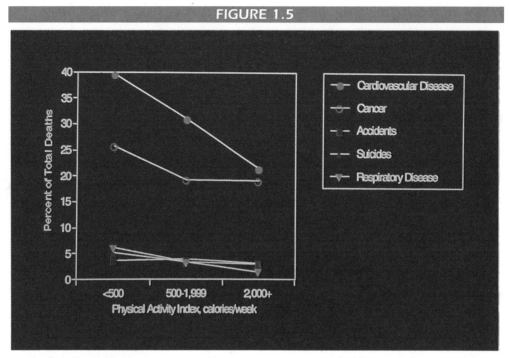

Cause-specific death rates[a] per 10,000 man-years of observation among Harvard alumni, 1962–1978, by physical activity index.

From Paffenbarger, R. S., R. T. Hyde, A. L. Wing, and C. H. Steinmetz. "A Natural History of Athleticism and Cardiovascular Health.' *JAMA* 252:491–495, 1985.

[a] Adjusted for differences in age, cigarette smoking, and hypertension.

the following list summarizes many of these benefits.

1. Improves and strengthens the cardio-vascular system (improved oxygen supply to all parts of the body, including the heart, the muscles, and the brain).

2. Maintains better muscle tone, muscular strength, and endurance.

3. Improves muscular flexibility.

4. Helps maintain recommended body weight.

5. Improves posture and physical appearance.

6. Decreases risk for chronic diseases and illness (coronary heart disease, cancer, and strokes, among others).

7. Lowers mortality rate from chronic diseases.

8. Thins the blood so it doesn't clot as readily (decreasing the risk for coronary heart disease and strokes).

9. Lowers blood pressure.

10. Helps prevent diabetes.

11. Enables people to sleep better.

12. Helps prevent chronic back pain.

FIGURE 1.6

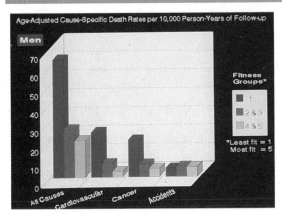
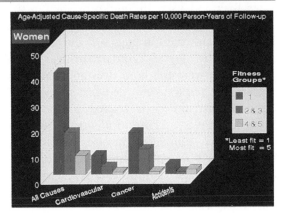

Age-adjusted cause-specific death rates per 10,000 person-years of follow-up (1970 to 1985) by physical fitness groups in men and women in the Aerobics Center longitudinal study in Dallas, Texas.

Based on data from Blair, S. N., H. W. Kohl III, R. S. Paffenbarger, Jr., D. G. Clark, K. H. Cooper, and L. W. Gibbons. "Physical Fitness and All-Cause Mortality: A Prospective Study of Healthy Men and Women." JAMA 262:2395–2401, 1989.

13. Relieves tension and helps in coping with stresses of life.

14. Increases levels of energy and job productivity.

15. Increases longevity and slows down the aging process.

16. Improves self-image and morale and aids in fighting depression.

17. Motivates toward positive lifestyle changes (better nutrition, smoking cessation, alcohol and drug abuse control).

18. Decreases recovery time following physical exertion.

19. Speeds up recovery following injury and/or disease.

20. Regulates and improves overall body functions.

21. Improves physical stamina and helps decrease chronic fatigue.

22. Eases the process of childbearing and childbirth.

23. Enhances quality of life; makes people feel better and live a healthier and happier life.

Fitness and Longevity

In addition to the benefits listed, research studies linking physical activity habits and mortality rates have shown a lower premature mortality rates in physically active people. Work conducted by Dr. Ralph Paffenbarger and colleagues, published in the *Journal of the American Medical Association* in 1985, demonstrated that as the amount of weekly physical activity increased, the risk of cardiovascular deaths decreased. In this study, conducted among 16,936 Harvard alumni, the greatest decrease in cardiovascular deaths was observed in alumni who burned more than 2,000 calories per week through physical activity (see Figure 1.5).

Another major study, conducted by Dr. Steve Blair and associates and published in the *Journal of the American Medical Association* in 1989, upheld the findings of the Harvard alumni study. Based on data from 13,344 people who were followed over an average of 8 years, the results confirmed that the level of cardiovascular fitness is related to mortality from all causes. These findings showed a graded and consistent inverse relationship between cardiovascular fitness and mortality, regardless of age and other risk factors. In essence, the higher the level of cardiovascular fitness, the longer the life (see Figure 1.6).

Death-rate from all causes for the least fit (group 1) men was 3.4 times higher than for the most fit men. For the least fit women, the death rate was 4.6 times higher than for the most fit women. The study also reported a greatly reduced rate of premature deaths, even at moderate fitness levels that most adults can easily achieve. People gain further protection when they combine higher fitness levels with reduction in other risk factors such as hypertension, elevated cholesterol, cigarette smoking, and excessive body fat.

THE PATH TO FITNESS AND BETTER QUALITY OF LIFE

Current scientific data and the fitness movement of the past two decades have led many people in the United States to see the advantages of participating in fitness programs that will improve and maintain adequate health. Because fitness and wellness needs vary significantly from one individual to another, all exercise and wellness prescriptions must be personalized for best results. This book provides the necessary guidelines for developing a lifetime program to improve fitness and promote preventive health care and personal wellness. As you study this book and complete the assignments in each chapter, you will learn to:

- Determine whether medical clearance is required for safe exercise participation.
- Assess your overall level of physical fitness, including cardiovascular endurance, muscular strength and endurance, muscular flexibility, and body composition.
- Prescribe personal programs for total fitness development.
- Write sound diet and weight control programs.
- Implement a healthy lifestyle program that includes prevention of cardiovascular diseases, cancer, stress management, and smoking cessation.
- Discern between myths and facts of exercise and health-related concepts.

GETTING STARTED

Even though exercise testing and participation are relatively safe for most apparently healthy individuals under age 40, a small but real risk exists for exercise-induced abnormalities in people with a history of cardiovascular problems and those who are at higher risk for disease. These people should be screened before initiating or increasing the intensity of an exercise program. Therefore, before you start an exercise program or participate in any exercise testing, you should fill out the health history questionnaire provided in Figure 1.7. A "yes" answer to any of these questions may signal a physician's approval before you participate. If you don't have any "yes" responses, you can proceed to Chapter 2 to assess your current level of fitness.

FIGURE 1.7

Health History Questionnaire

Even though exercise participation is relatively safe for most apparently healthy individuals, the reaction of the cardiovascular system to increased levels of physical activity cannot always be totally predicted. Consequently, there is a small but real risk of certain changes occurring during exercise participation. These changes may include abnormal blood pressure, irregular heart rhythm, fainting, and in rare instances a heart attack or cardiac arrest. Therefore, you must provide honest answers to this questionnaire. Exercise may not be recommended under some of the conditions listed below; others may simply indicate special consideration. If any of the conditions apply, you should consult your physician before participating in an exercise program. You also should promptly report to your instructor any exercise-related abnormalities experienced during the course of the semester.

Have you ever had or do you now have any of the following conditions?

☐ Yes ☐ No   1. Cardiovascular disease (any type of heart or blood vessel disease, including strokes)

☐ Yes ☐ No   2. Elevated blood lipids (cholesterol and triglycerides)

☐ Yes ☐ No   3. Chest pain at rest or during exertion

☐ Yes ☐ No   4. Shortness of breath or other respiratory problems

☐ Yes ☐ No   5. Uneven, irregular, or skipped heartbeats (including a racing or fluttering heart)

☐ Yes ☐ No   6. Elevated blood pressure

☐ Yes ☐ No   7. Often feel faint or have spells of severe dizziness

☐ Yes ☐ No   8. Diabetes

☐ Yes ☐ No   9. Any joint, bone, or muscle problems (e.g., arthritis, low back pain, rheumatism)

☐ Yes ☐ No 10. An eating disorder (anorexia, bulimia)

☐ Yes ☐ No 11. Any other concern regarding your ability to safely participate in an exercise program? If so, explain:

Indicate if any of the following two conditions apply:

☐ Yes ☐ No 12. Do you smoke cigarettes?

☐ Yes ☐ No 13. Men — Are you age 40 or older?

☐ Yes ☐ No 14. Women — Are you age 50 or older?

Student's Signature: _____ Date: _____

Physical Fitness Assessment

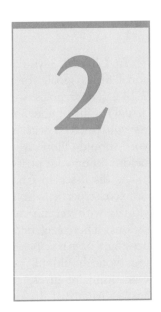

KEY CONCEPTS

- Health fitness standards
- Physical fitness standards
- Cardiovascular endurance
- Aerobic fitness
- Maximal oxygen uptake
- Resting metabolic rate
- Muscular strength
- Muscular endurance
- One repetition maximum
- Muscular flexibility
- Body composition
- Percent body fat
- Lean body mass
- Essential fat
- Storage fat

OBJECTIVES

- Define the health-related components of physical fitness.
- Be able to assess cardiovascular fitness, strength fitness, flexibility fitness, and body composition.
- Be able to determine recommended body weight.

The health-related components of physical fitness include cardiovascular endurance, muscular strength and endurance, muscular flexibility, and body composition. These four components are the topics of this chapter, along with basic techniques frequently used in their assessment. Through these assessment techniques, you will be able to regularly determine your physical fitness level as you engage in an exercise program. You are encouraged to conduct fitness assessments at least twice — once as a pre-test, which will serve as a starting point, and later as a post-test, to assess improvements in fitness following 10 to 14 weeks of exercise participation.

A personal fitness profile is provided in Figure A.1, Appendix A, for you to record the results of each fitness assessment in this chapter (pre-test). Figure A.2 can be used at the end of the term to record the results of your post-test.*

*You may obtain a computerized fitness profile by using the software for this book available to your instructor from Morton Publishing Company, 925 W. Kenyon, Unit 12, Englewood, Colorado 80110. An example of the a profile is given in Figure A.3.

In Chapter 3 you will learn to write personal fitness goals for this course (see Figure 3.14). These goals should be based on the actual results of your initial fitness assessments. As you proceed with your exercise program, you should allow a minimum of 8 weeks before doing your post-fitness assessments.

As discussed in Chapter 1, exercise testing or exercise participation is not advised for individuals with certain medical or physical conditions. Therefore, before starting an exercise program or participating in any exercise testing, you should fill out the Health History Questionnaire given in Figure 1.7. A "yes" answer to any of the questions signals consultation with a physician before initiating, continuing, or increasing your level of physical activity.

PHYSICAL FITNESS ASSESSMENT

No single test can provide a complete measure of physical fitness. Because fitness has four different components, a battery of tests is necessary to determine an individual's overall level of fitness.

In the next few pages are several tests used to assess the health-related fitness components. When interpreting fitness test results, *two standards can be applied: health fitness and physical fitness.*

The proposed *health fitness standards* are based on epidemiological* data linking minimum fitness values to health and disease prevention. These standards seem to be the lowest fitness requirements to maintain good health, lessen the risk for chronic diseases, and reduce the incidence of muscular-skeletal injuries. Attaining the health fitness standards requires only moderate amounts of physical activity. For example, a 2-mile walking

---

*Epidemiology is the study of diseases that affect many individuals within a population.

program in less than 30 minutes, five to six times per week, seems to be sufficient to achieve the health fitness standard for cardiovascular endurance.

Physical fitness standards are usually set higher than the health fitness norms and require a more vigorous exercise program. Many experts believe that people who meet the criteria of "good" physical fitness should be able to perform moderate to vigorous amounts of physical activity without undue fatigue and also maintain this capability throughout life. In this context, physically fit people of all ages have the freedom to enjoy most of life's daily and recreational activities to their fullest potential. Current health fitness standards may not be enough to achieve these objectives.

For the purposes of this book, both health fitness and physical fitness standards are given for each fitness test. The individual has to decide the objectives of the fitness program. If the main objective of the fitness program is to decrease the risk for disease, meeting the health fitness standards may suffice to ensure better health. On the other hand, if the individual wants to participate in moderate to vigorous fitness activities, attaining a high physical fitness standard is recommended.

CARDIOVASCULAR ENDURANCE

Cardiovascular endurance has been defined as *the ability of the lungs, heart, and blood vessels to deliver adequate amounts of oxygen to the cells to meet the demands of prolonged physical activity.* As a person breathes, part of the oxygen in the air is taken up in the lungs and transported in the blood to the heart. The heart then pumps the oxygenated blood through the circulatory system to all organs and tissues of the body. At the cellular level, oxygen is used to convert food substrates, primarily carbohydrates and fats, into the energy necessary to conduct body functions, maintain a constant internal equilibrium, and perform physical tasks.

Some examples of activities that promote cardiovascular or aerobic fitness are walking, jogging, cycling, rowing, swimming, cross-country skiing, aerobics, soccer, basketball, and racquetball (see Figure 2.1). The necessary guidelines to develop a lifetime cardiovascular endurance exercise program are given in Chapter 3 and an introduction and description of benefits of leading aerobic activities are given in Chapter 4.

A sound cardiovascular endurance program greatly contributes to good health. The typical American is not exactly a good role model

FIGURE 2.1

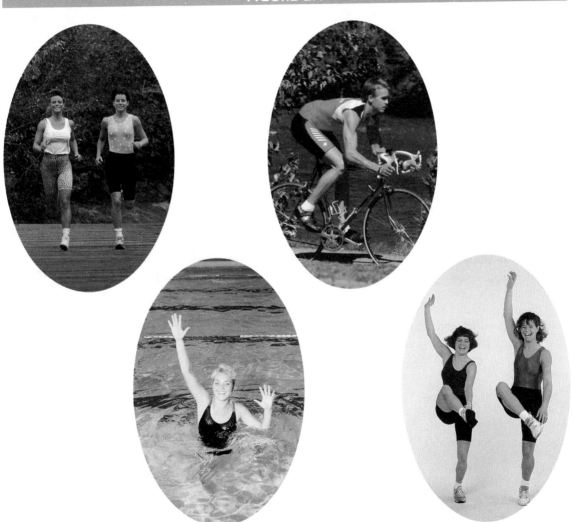

Aerobic activities promote cardiovascular development and help decrease the risk for chronic diseases.

when physical fitness is concerned. A poorly conditioned heart that has to pump more often just to keep a person alive is subject to more wear-and-tear than a well-conditioned heart is. In situations that place strenuous demands on the heart, such as doing yard work, lifting heavy objects or weights, or running to catch a bus, the unconditioned heart may not be able to sustain the strain.

Everyone who initiates a cardiovascular exercise program can expect a number of benefits from training. Among these are lower resting heart rate, blood pressure, blood lipids (cholesterol and triglycerides), recovery time following exercise, and risk for hypokinetic diseases (those associated with physical inactivity and sedentary living). Simultaneously, cardiac muscle strength and oxygen-carrying capacity increases.

Cardiovascular endurance is determined by the maximal amount of oxygen (maximal oxygen uptake or VO_{2max}) the human body is able to utilize per minute of physical activity. The VO_{2max} usually is expressed in ml/kg/min. Because all tissues and organs of the body utilize oxygen to function, more oxygen consumption means a more efficient cardiovascular system.

During physical exertion, more energy is needed to perform the activity. As a result, the heart, lungs, and blood vessels have to deliver more oxygen to the cells to supply the required energy. During prolonged exercise, an individual with a high level of cardiovascular endurance is able to deliver the required amount of oxygen to the tissues with relative ease. The cardiovascular system of a person with a low level of endurance has to work much harder, as the heart has to pump more often to supply the same amount of oxygen to the tissues and consequently fatigues faster. Hence, a higher capacity to deliver and utilize oxygen (oxygen uptake) indicates a more efficient cardiovascular system.

Even though most cardiovascular endurance tests are probably safe to administer to apparently healthy individuals (those with no major coronary risk factors or symptoms), the American College of Sports Medicine recommends that a physician be present for all maximal exercise tests on apparently healthy men over age 40 and women over 50. A maximal test is any test that requires the participant's all-out or nearly all-out effort, such as the 1.5-mile run test or a maximal exercise stress test (see Figure 2.2). For submaximal exercise tests (such as a walking test), a physician should be present when testing higher risk/symptomatic individuals or people with medical conditions, regardless of the participant's age.

FIGURE 2.2

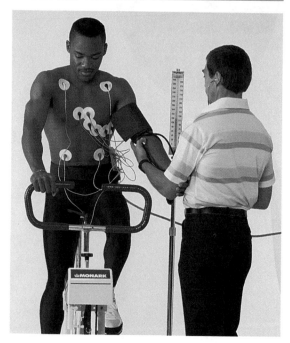

Exercise tolerance test with twelve-lead electrocardiographic monitoring (stress ECG).

The 1.5-Mile Run Test

The test used most often to determine cardiovascular fitness is the 1.5-mile run test. The fitness category is determined according to the time a person takes to run or walk a 1.5-mile course. The only equipment necessary to conduct this test is a stopwatch and a track or premeasured 1.5-mile course.

The 1.5-mile run test is quite simple to administer, but it requires caution. Because the objective of the test is to cover the distance in the shortest time, this test is for conditioned individuals who have been cleared for exercise. It is not recommended for unconditioned beginners, symptomatic individuals, those with known cardiovascular disease or heart disease risk factors, and men over age 40 and women over 50. Unconditioned beginners are encouraged to have at least 6 weeks of aerobic training before they take the test.

Prior to taking the 1.5-mile run test you should do a few warm-up exercises — some stretching exercises, some walking, and slow jogging. Next, time yourself during the 1.5-mile run to see how fast you cover the distance. If any unusual symptoms arise during the test, do not continue. Stop immediately and see your physician or retake the test after another 6 weeks of aerobic training. At the end of the test, cool down by walking or jogging slowly for another 3 to 5 minutes. Referring to your performance time, look up your estimated VO_{2max} in Table 2.1 and the corresponding fitness category in Table 2.2.

TABLE 2.1

Estimated Maximal Oxygen Uptake in ml/kg/min for the 1.5-mile Run Test.

Time	Max VO$_2$	Time	Max VO$_2$	Time	Max VO$_2$	Time	Max VO$_2$
6:10	80.0	9:30	54.7	12:50	39.2	16:10	30.5
6:20	79.0	9:40	53.5	13:00	38.6	16:20	30.2
6:30	77.9	9:50	52.3	13:10	38.1	16:30	29.8
6:40	76.7	10:00	51.1	13:20	37.8	16:40	29.5
6:50	75.5	10:10	50.4	13:30	37.2	16:50	29.1
7:00	74.0	10:20	49.5	13:40	36.8	17:00	28.9
7:10	72.6	10:30	48.6	13:50	36.3	17:10	28.5
7:20	71.3	10:40	48.0	14:00	35.9	17:20	28.3
7:30	69.9	10:50	47.4	14:10	35.5	17:30	28.0
7:40	68.3	11:00	46.6	14:20	35.1	17:40	27.7
7:50	66.8	11:10	45.8	14:30	34.7	17:50	27.4
8:00	65.2	11:20	45.1	14:40	34.3	18:00	27.1
8:10	63.9	11:30	44.4	14:50	34.0	18:10	26.8
8:20	62.5	11:40	43.7	15:00	33.6	18:20	26.6
8:30	61.2	11:50	43.2	15:10	33.1	18:30	26.3
8:40	60.2	12:00	42.3	15:20	32.7	18:40	26.0
8:50	59.1	12:10	41.7	15:30	32.2	18:50	25.7
9:00	58.1	12:20	41.0	15:40	31.8	19:00	25.4
9:10	56.9	12:30	40.4	15:50	31.4		
9:20	55.9	12:40	39.8	16:00	30.9		

Adapted from Cooper, K. H. "A Means of Assessing Maximal Oxygen Intake." *JAMA* 203:201-204, 1968; Pollock, M. L. et. al. *Health and Fitness Through Physical Activity.* New York: John Wiley and Sons, 1978: Wilmore, J. H. *Training for Sport and Activity.* Boston: Allyn and Bacon, 1982.

TABLE 2.2

Cardiovascular fitness classification according to maximal oxygen uptake ($VO_{2 max}$) in milliliters per kilogram per minute (ml/kg/min.)

| Gender | Age | Fitness Classification | | | | |
		Poor	Fair	Average	Good	Excellent
Men	≤29	≤24	25–33	34–43	44–52	≥53
	30–39	≤22	23–30	31–41	42–49	≥50
	40–49	≤19	20–26	27–38	39–44	≥45
	50–59	≤17	18–24	25–37	38–42	≥43
	60–69	≤15	16–22	23–35	36–40	≥41
Women	≤29	≤23	24–30	31–38	39–48	≥49
	30–39	≤19	20–27	28–36	37–44	≥45
	40–49	≤16	17–24	25–34	35–41	≥42
	50–59	≤14	15–21	22–33	34–39	≥40
	60–69	≤12	13–20	21–32	33–36	≥37

■ High physical fitness standard

■ Health fitness standard

For example, a 20-year-old female runs the 1.5-mile course in 12 minutes and 40 seconds. Table 2.1 shows a VO_{2max} of 39.8 ml/kg/min. for a time of 12:40. According to Table 2.2, this VO_{2max} would place her in the good cardiovascular fitness category.

The 1.0-Mile Walk Test*

The walking test calls for a 440-yard track (four laps to a mile) or a premeasured 1.0-mile course. Body weight in pounds must be determined prior to the walk. A stopwatch is required to measure total walking time and exercise heart rate.

You can proceed to walk the 1.0-mile course at a brisk pace so that the exercise heart rate at the end of the test is above 120 beats per minute. At the end of the 1.0-mile walk, check your walking time and immediately

count your pulse for 10 seconds. You can take your pulse on the wrist by placing two fingers over the radial artery (inside of the wrist on the side of the thumb) or over the carotid artery in the neck just below the jaw next to the voice box (see Figures 2.3 and 2.4).

FIGURE 2.3

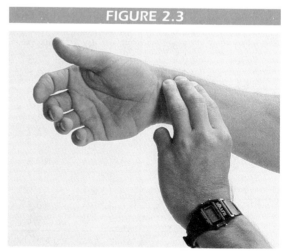

Pulse taken at the radial artery.

*Source: Kline, G. et al., 1987, "Estimation of VO_{2max} from a One-Mile Track Walk, Gender, Age, and Body Weight," *Medicine and Science in Sports and Exercise* 19(3):253-259, 1987. © American College of Sports Medicine.

FIGURE 2.4

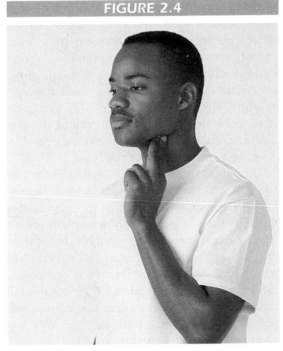

Pulse taken at the carotid artery.

Next multiply the 10-second pulse count by 6 to obtain the exercise heart rate in beats per minute. Now convert the walking time from minutes and seconds to minute units. Each minute has 60 seconds, so the seconds are divided by 60 to obtain the fraction of a minute. For instance, a walking time of 12 minutes and 15 seconds would equal 12 + (15 ÷ 60) or 12.25 minutes.

To obtain the estimated VO_{2max} in ml/kg/min. for the 1.0-mile walk test, plug your values in the following equation:

$$VO_{2max} = 132.853 - (.0769 \times W) - (.3877 \times A) + (6.315 \times G) - (3.2649 \times T) - (.1565 \times HR)$$

where:

W = Weight in pounds
A = Age in years

G = Gender; use 0 for women and 1 for men
T = Total time for the one-mile walk in minutes
HR = Exercise heart rate in beats per minute at the end of the one-mile walk

For example, a 19-year-old female subject who weighs 140 pounds completed the one-mile walk in 14 minutes and 39 seconds and with an exercise heart rate of 148 beats per minute. The estimated VO_{2max} would be:

W = 140 lbs
A = 19
G = 0 (female gender)
T = 14:39 = 14 + (39 ÷ 60) = 14.65 min.
HR = 148 bpm

$$VO_{2max} = 132.853 - (.0769 \times 140) - (.3877 \times 19) + (6.315 \times 0) - (3.2649 \times 14.65) - (.1565 \times 148)$$

$$VO_{2max} = 43.7 \text{ ml/kg/min.}$$

As with the 1.5-mile run test, the fitness categories based on VO_{2max} are found in Table 2.2. Be sure to record your cardiovascular fitness test results on your fitness profile in Figure A.1.

MUSCULAR STRENGTH/ENDURANCE

Many people are under the impression that muscular strength and endurance are necessary only for athletes and others who hold jobs that require heavy muscular work. Strength and endurance, however, are important components of total physical fitness and have become essential to everyone's life.

Adequate levels of strength significantly enhance a person's health and well-being throughout life. Strength is crucial for top performance in daily activities such as sitting, walking, running, lifting and carrying objects, doing housework, and even enjoying recreational activities. Strength is also valuable in improving personal appearance and self-image, developing sports skills, and meeting certain emergencies in life where strength is necessary to cope effectively.

Perhaps one of the most significant benefits of maintaining a good strength level is its relationship to human *metabolism* — all energy and material transformations that take place within living cells. A primary result of a strength training program is an increase in muscle mass or size, known as *muscle hypertrophy.*

Muscle tissue uses energy even at rest, whereas fatty tissue uses very little energy and may be considered metabolically inert from the standpoint of caloric use. As muscle size increases, so does resting metabolism or the amount of energy (expressed in milliliters of oxygen per minute or total calories per day) an individual requires during resting conditions to sustain proper body function. Even small increases in muscle mass may affect resting metabolism. Each additional pound of muscle tissue increases resting metabolism by an estimated 30 to 50 calories per day. All other factors being equal, if two individuals who weigh 150 pounds each but have different amounts of muscle mass, let's say 5 pounds, the one with the greater muscle mass will have a higher resting metabolic rate, allowing this person to eat more calories to maintain the muscle tissue.

Although muscular strength and endurance are interrelated, there is a basic difference between the two. *Muscular strength is the ability to exert maximum force against resistance. Muscular endurance is the ability of a muscle to exert submaximal force repeatedly over a period of time.* Muscular endurance (also called localized muscular endurance) depends to a large extent on muscular strength and to a lesser extent on cardiovascular endurance. Weak muscles cannot repeat an action several times or sustain it for long. Keeping these concepts in mind, strength tests and training programs have been designed to measure and develop absolute muscular strength, muscular endurance, or a combination of the two.

Muscular strength usually is determined by the maximal amount of resistance (one repetition maximum, or 1 RM) that a person is able to lift in a single effort. This assessment gives a good measure of absolute strength, but it does require a considerable amount of time to administer. Muscular endurance is commonly established by the number of repetitions an individual can perform against a submaximal resistance or by the length of time a person can sustain a given contraction.

Muscular Endurance Test

We live in a world in which muscular strength and endurance are both required, and muscular endurance depends to a large extent on muscular strength. Accordingly, a muscular endurance test has been selected to determine strength level. Three exercises that help assess endurance of the upper body, lower body, and abdominal/hip flexors muscle groups have been selected for your muscular endurance test. You will need a stopwatch, a metronome, a bench or gymnasium bleacher 16¼ inches high, and a partner to perform the test.

The exercises conducted for this test are bench-jumps, modified-dips (men) or modified push-ups (women), and bent-leg curl-ups. All exercises should be conducted with the aid of a partner. The correct procedures for performing each exercise follow.

Bench-Jumps

Using a bench or gymnasium bleacher 16¼ inches high, attempt to jump up and down on the bench as many times as you can in a 1-minute period (see Figure 2.5). If you cannot jump the full minute, you may step up and down. A repetition is counted each time both feet return to the floor.

FIGURE 2.5

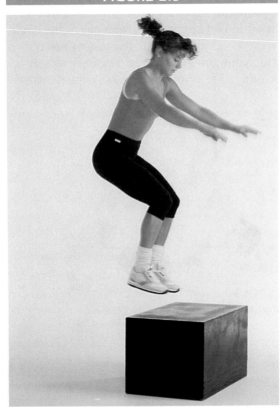

Bench-jumps.

Modified-Dip

This upper-body exercise is done by men only. Using a bench or gymnasium bleacher, place your hands on the bench with the fingers pointing forward. Have a partner hold your feet in front of you. The hips should be bent at approximately 90 degrees (you also may use three sturdy chairs; put your hands on two chairs placed by the sides of your body and your feet on the third chair in front of you).

Next, lower the body by flexing the elbows until you reach a 90-degree angle at this joint, and then return to the starting position (see Figure 2.6). The repetition does not count if you fail to reach 90 degrees. The repetitions are performed to a two-step cadence (down-up), regulated with a metronome set at 56 beats per minute. Perform as many continuous repetitions as possible. You can no longer count the repetitions if you fail to follow the metronome cadence.

FIGURE 2.6

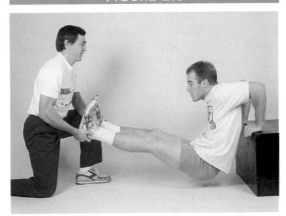

Modified-dip.

Modified Push-Ups

Women perform the modified push-up exercise instead of the chair-dip exercise. Lie down on the floor (face down), bend the knees (feet up in the air), and place the hands on the floor by the shoulders with the fingers pointing forward. The lower body will be supported at the knees (rather than the feet) throughout the test (see Figure 2.7). The chest must touch the floor on each repetition.

FIGURE 2.7

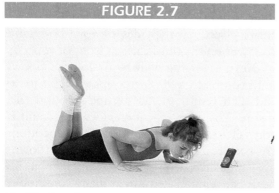

Modified push-ups.

As with the chair-dip exercise, the repetitions are performed to a two-step cadence (up-down) regulated with a metronome set at 56 beats per minute. Do as many continuous repetitions as possible. You cannot count any more repetitions if you fail to follow the metronome cadence.

Bent-Leg Curl-Ups

Lie down on the floor (face up) and bend both legs at the knees at approximately 100 degrees. Feet should be on the floor, and you must hold them in place yourself throughout the test. Cross the arms in front of your chest, each hand on the opposite shoulder.

Now raise your head off the floor, placing the chin against your chest. This is the starting and finishing position for each curl-up (see Figure 2.8). The back of the head may not come in contact with the floor, the hands cannot be removed from the shoulders, and the feet or hips may not be raised off the floor at any time during the test. The test is terminated if any of these four conditions occur.

When you curl-up, the upper body must come to an upright position before going back down (see Figure 2.9). The repetitions are performed to a two-step cadence (up-down) regulated with the metronome set at 40 beats

per minute. For this exercise, allow a brief practice period of 10 to 15 seconds to familiarize yourself with the cadence. **Initiate the up movement with the first beat, then wait for the next beat to initiate the down movement. One repetition is accomplished every two beats of the metronome.**

Count as many repetitions as you are able to do following the proper cadence. This test, too, is terminated if you do not maintain the appropriate cadence or if you complete 100 repetitions. Have your partner check the angle at the knees throughout the test to make sure you maintain 100-degree angle as closely as possible. Perform this test on a gym mat or

FIGURE 2.8

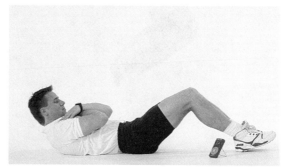

Starting position for bent-leg curl-ups.

FIGURE 2.9

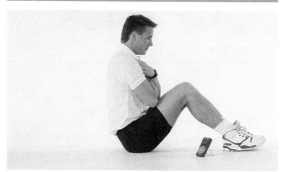

Upright position for bent-leg curl-ups.

similar surface to prevent bruising of the coccyx (tailbone) area.

According to your results, look up your percentile rank for each exercise in the far left column of Table 2.3. Next, total the percentile scores for each exercise, and divide by 3 to obtain an average score. You can determine your individual and overall muscular endurance fitness categories according to the ratings in Table 2.4.

TABLE 2.3

Muscular Endurance Scoring

MEN

Percentile Rank	Bench Jumps	Modified Dips	Bent-leg Curl-ups
99	66	54	100
95	63	50	81
90	62	38	65
80	58	32	51
70	57	30	44
60	56	27	31
50	54	26	28
40	51	23	25
30	48	20	22
20	47	17	17
10	40	11	10
5	34	7	3

WOMEN

Percentile Rank	Bench Jumps	Modified Push-ups	Bent-leg Curl-ups
99	58	95	100+
95	54	70	100
90	52	50	97
80	48	41	77
70	44	38	57
60	42	33	45
50	39	30	37
40	38	28	28
30	36	25	22
20	32	21	17
10	28	18	9
5	26	15	4

High physical fitness standard

Health fitness standard

*Reproduced with permission from Hoeger, W.W.K. *Principles and Labs for Physical Fitness & Wellness.* Morton Publishing Company, Englewood, Colorado, 1991.

TABLE 2.4

Fitness Categories Based on Percentile Ranks

Average Score	Endurance Classification
≥81	Excellent
61–80	Good
41–60	Average
21–40	Fair
≤20	Poor

High physical fitness standard

Health fitness standard

MUSCULAR FLEXIBILITY

Flexibility is the ability of a joint to move freely through its full range of motion. Total range of motion around a joint is highly specific and varies from one joint to the other (hip, trunk, shoulder), as well as from one individual to the next. Muscular flexibility relates primarily to genetic factors and index of physical activity. Beyond that, factors such as joint structure, ligaments, tendons, muscles, skin, tissue injury, adipose tissue (fat), body temperature, age, and gender influence range of motion about a joint.

On the average, women have higher flexibility levels than men and seem to retain this advantage throughout life. Aging decreases the extensibility of soft tissue, decreasing flexibility in both genders. The most significant contributors to a loss in flexibility, however, are sedentary living and lack of physical activity.

Developing and maintaining some level of flexibility are important in all health enhancement programs, and even more so during the aging process. Sports medicine specialists say that many muscular/skeletal problems and injuries, especially in adults, are related to a lack of flexibility.

Most experts agree that participating in a regular flexibility program will help a person maintain good joint mobility, increase resistance to muscle injury and soreness, prevent low back and other spinal column problems, improve and maintain good postural alignment, enhance proper and graceful body movement, improve personal appearance and self-image, and facilitate motor skills throughout life. Flexibility exercises also have been used successfully in treating patients with dysmenorrhea and general neuromuscular tension. Stretching exercises in conjunction with calisthenics are helpful in warm-up routines to prepare for more vigorous aerobic or strength-training exercises, as well as subsequent cool-down routines to help return to the normal resting state.

Flexibility Assessment

Two flexibility tests are used to determine your flexibility profile. These are the modified sit-and-reach test and the total body rotation test.

Modified Sit-and-Reach Test

To perform this test you will need the Acuflex I* sit-and-reach flexibility tester or you may simply place a yardstick on top of a

*The Acuflex I and II flexibility testers for the modified sit-and-reach and the total body rotation tests can be obtained from Novel Products Figure Finder Collection, P.O. Box 408, Rockton, IL 61072-0408, (800) 624-4888.

box approximately 12 inches high. The procedure to administer this test is:

1. Be sure to properly warm up before the first trial.

2. Remove your shoes for the test. Sit on the floor with your hips, back, and head against a wall, legs fully extended, and the bottom of the feet against the Acuflex I or the sit-and-reach box.

3. Place the hands one on top of the other and reach forward as far as possible without letting the hips, back, or head come off the wall. Another person then should slide the reach indicator on the Acuflex I (or yardstick) along the top of the box until the end of the indicator touches the tips of your fingers (see Figure 2.10). The indicator must be held firmly in place throughout the rest of the test.

4. The head and back now can come off the wall and you may gradually reach forward three times, the third time stretching forward as far as possible on the indicator (or

FIGURE 2.10

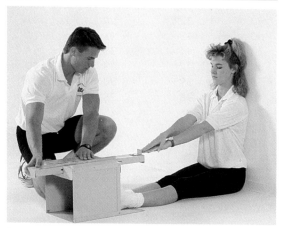

Determining the starting position for the modified sit-and-reach test.

yardstick), holding the final position for at least 2 seconds (see Figure 2.11). Be sure to keep the back of the knees against the floor throughout the test. Record the final

FIGURE 2.11

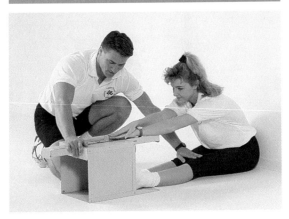

The modified sit-and-reach test.

number of inches reached to the nearest half inch.

5. You are allowed two trials and an average of the two scores is used as the final test score. The percentile ranks and fitness categories for this test are given in Tables 2.5 and 2.4, respectively.

Total Body Rotation Test

An Acuflex II total body rotation flexibility tester or a measuring scale with a sliding panel is needed to administer this test. The Acuflex II or scale is placed on the wall at shoulder height and should be adjustable to accommodate individual differences in height.

If no sliding panel is available, you can build your own scale. Glue or tape a measuring tape above the sliding panel and another below it — centered at the 15-inch mark. Each tape should be at least 30 inches long.

TABLE 2.5

Percentile Ranks for the Modified Sit-and-Reach Test*

	Percentile Rank	Age Category					Percentile	Age Category			
		<18	19–35	36–49	50>			<18	19–35	36–49	50>
	99	20.8	20.1	18.9	16.2		99	22.6	21.0	19.8	17.2
	95	19.6	18.9	18.2	15.8		95	19.5	19.3	19.2	15.7
	90	18.2	17.2	16.1	15.0		90	18.7	17.9	17.4	15.0
	80	17.8	17.0	14.6	13.3		80	17.8	16.7	16.2	14.2
	70	16.0	15.8	13.9	12.3		70	16.5	16.2	15.2	13.6
	60	15.2	15.0	13.4	11.5		60	16.0	15.8	14.5	12.3
Men	50	14.5	14.4	12.6	10.2	Women	50	15.2	14.8	13.5	11.1
	40	14.0	13.5	11.6	9.7		40	14.5	14.5	12.8	10.1
	30	13.4	13.0	10.8	9.3		30	13.7	13.7	12.2	9.2
	20	11.8	11.6	9.9	8.8		20	12.6	12.6	11.0	8.3
	10	9.5	9.2	8.3	7.8		10	11.4	10.1	9.7	7.5
	05	8.4	7.9	7.0	7.2		05	9.4	8.1	8.5	3.7
	01	7.2	7.0	5.1	4.0		01	6.5	2.6	2.0	1.5

▨ High physical fitness standard

▇ Health fitness standard

*Reproduced with permission from Hoeger, W.W.K. *Lifetime Physical Fitness & Wellness: A Personalized Program.* Englewood, CO: Morton Publishing Company, 1992.

Draw a line on the floor, centered with the 15-inch mark (see Figures 2.12, 2.13, 2.14, and 2.15). Use the following procedure:

1. Properly warm up before beginning this test.

FIGURE 2.15

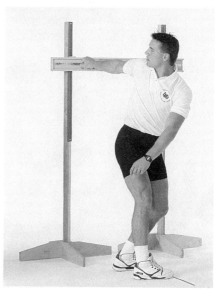

Total body rotation test.

FIGURE 2.12

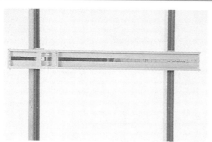

Acuflex II measuring device for the total body rotation test.

FIGURE 2.13

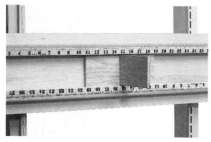

Homemade measuring device for the total body rotation test.

FIGURE 2.14

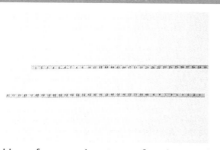

Use of measuring tapes for the total body rotation test.

2. To start, stand sideways, an arm's length away from the wall, with the feet straight ahead, slightly separated, and the toes right up to the corresponding line drawn on the floor. Hold out the arm opposite the wall horizontally from the body, making a fist. The Acuflex II, measuring scale, or tapes should be shoulder height at this time.

3. Now rotate the body, the extended arm going backward (always maintaining a horizontal plane) and making contact with the panel, gradually sliding it forward as far as possible. If no panel is available, slide the fist alongside the tapes as far as possible. Hold the final position at least 2 seconds.

   Position the hand with the little finger side forward during the entire sliding movement, as illustrated in Figure 2.16. **The proper hand position is crucial. Some people attempt to open the hand or push with extended fingers or slide the panel with the knuckles, none of**

FIGURE 2.16

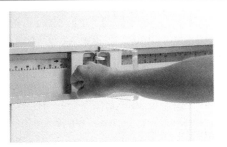

Proper hand position for the total body rotation test.

which is acceptable. During the test, the knees can be slightly bent, but **the feet cannot be moved; they always must point straight forward.** The body must be kept as straight (vertical) as possible.

4. Conduct the test on either the right or the left side of the body. Two trials are allowed on the selected side. The farthest point reached, measured to the nearest half inch and held for at least 2 seconds, is recorded. The average of the two trials is the final test score. Referring to Tables 2.6 and 2.4, you

TABLE 2.6

Percentile Ranks for the Total Body Rotation Test*

	Percentile Rank	Left Rotation				Right Rotation			
		<18	19–35	36–49	50>	<18	19–35	36–49	50>
Men	99	29.1	28.0	26.6	21.0	28.2	27.8	25.2	22.2
	95	26.6	24.8	24.5	20.0	25.5	25.6	23.8	20.7
	90	25.0	23.6	23.0	17.7	24.3	24.1	22.5	19.3
	80	22.0	22.0	21.2	15.5	22.7	22.3	21.0	16.3
	70	20.9	20.3	20.4	14.7	21.3	20.7	18.7	15.7
	60	19.9	19.3	18.7	13.9	19.8	19.0	17.3	14.7
	50	18.6	18.0	16.7	12.7	19.0	17.2	16.3	12.3
	40	17.0	16.8	15.3	11.7	17.3	16.3	14.7	11.5
	30	14.9	15.0	14.8	10.3	15.1	15.0	13.3	10.7
	20	13.8	13.3	13.7	9.5	12.9	13.3	11.2	8.7
	10	10.8	10.5	10.8	4.3	10.8	11.3	8.0	2.7
	05	8.5	8.9	8.8	0.3	8.1	8.3	5.5	0.3
	01	3.4	1.7	5.1	0.0	6.6	2.9	2.0	0.0
Women	99	29.3	28.6	27.1	23.0	29.6	29.4	27.1	21.7
	95	26.8	24.8	25.3	21.4	27.6	25.3	25.9	19.7
	90	25.5	23.0	23.4	20.5	25.8	23.0	21.3	19.0
	80	23.8	21.5	20.2	19.1	23.7	20.8	19.6	17.9
	70	21.8	20.5	18.6	17.3	22.0	19.3	17.3	16.8
	60	20.5	19.3	17.7	16.0	20.8	18.0	16.5	15.6
	50	19.5	18.0	16.4	14.8	19.5	17.3	14.6	14.0
	40	18.5	17.2	14.8	13.7	18.3	16.0	13.1	12.8
	30	17.1	15.7	13.6	10.0	16.3	15.2	11.7	8.5
	20	16.0	15.2	11.6	6.3	14.5	14.0	9.8	3.9
	10	12.8	13.6	8.5	3.0	12.4	11.1	6.1	2.2
	05	11.1	7.3	6.8	0.7	10.2	8.8	4.0	1.1
	01	8.9	5.3	4.3	0.0	8.9	3.2	2.8	0.0

▓ High physical fitness standard   ■ Health fitness standard

*Reproduced with permission from Hoeger, W.W.K. *Lifetime Physical Fitness & Wellness: A Personalized Program.* Englewood, CO: Morton Publishing Company, 1992.

can determine the respective percentile rank and flexibility fitness classification for this test.

After obtaining your score and percentile rank for both tests, you can determine the overall flexibility fitness classification by computing an average percentile rank from the two tests under the same guidelines as given in Table 2.4.

BODY COMPOSITION

Body composition refers to the fat and nonfat components of the human body. The fat component usually is called *fat mass* or *percent body fat*. The nonfat component is termed *lean body mass*.

For many years people have relied on height/weight charts to determine recommended body weight, but we now know that these tables can be highly inaccurate for many people. The standard height/weight tables, first published in 1912, were based on average weights (including shoes and clothing) for men and women who obtained life insurance policies between 1888 and 1905. The recommended weight on height/weight tables is obtained according to gender, height, and frame size. As no scientific guidelines are given to determine frame size, most people choose their frame size based on the column where the weight comes closest to their own.

The proper way to determine recommended weight is by finding out what percent of total body weight is fat and what amount is lean tissue (body composition). Once the fat percentage is known, recommended body weight, at which there is no harm to human health, can be calculated from recommended body fat.

The importance of good body composition in achieving and maintaining good health cannot be underestimated. Obesity is a health

hazard of epidemic proportions in most developed countries around the world. Obesity by itself has been associated with several serious health problems and accounts for 15 to 20% of the annual U.S. mortality rate. Obesity is a major risk factor for diseases of the cardiovascular system, including coronary heart disease, hypertension, congestive heart failure, elevated blood lipids, atherosclerosis, strokes, thromboembolitic disease, varicose veins, and intermittent claudication.

Almost everyone agrees that obese people have a higher mortality rate than those who are not obese, and scientific evidence also points out that the same is true for underweight people. Although the social pressure to be thin has waned slightly in recent years, pressure to attain model-like thinness is still with us and contributes to the gradual increase in eating disorders (anorexia nervosa and bulimia, discussed in Chapter 5). Extreme weight loss can spawn medical conditions such as heart damage, gastrointestinal problems, shrinkage of internal organs, immune system abnormalities, disorders of the reproductive system, loss of muscle tissue, damage to the nervous system, and even death.

To determine whether people are truly obese or not, body composition must be established. Obesity is related to an excess of body fat. If body weight is the only criterion, an individual can easily be overweight according to height/weight charts, yet not be obese. Football players, body builders, weight lifters, and other athletes with large muscle size are typical examples. Some of these athletes who appear to be 20 or 30 pounds overweight really have little body fat.

At the other end of the spectrum, some people who weigh very little and are viewed by many as "skinny" or underweight actually can be classified as overweight because of their high body fat content. People who weigh as little as 100 to 120 pounds but are more than

30% fat (about a third of their total body weight) are not uncommon. These people are often sedentary or constantly dieting. Physical inactivity and constant negative caloric balance both lead to a loss in lean body mass (see Chapter 5). Body weight alone clearly does not always tell the true story.

Total fat in the human body is classified into two types: essential fat and storage fat. Essential fat is needed for normal physiological functions. Without it, human health deteriorates. This essential fat constitutes about 3% of the total fat in men and 12% in women. The percentage is higher in women because it includes gender-specific fat, such as that found in the breast tissue, the uterus, and other gender-related fat deposits. *Storage fat* is the fat stored in adipose tissue, mostly beneath the skin (subcutaneous fat) and around major organs in the body.

Body Composition Assessment Through Skinfold Thickness

Assessment of body composition is most frequently done using skinfold thickness. This technique is based on the principle that approximately half of the body's fatty tissue is directly beneath the skin. Valid and reliable estimates of this tissue give a good indication of percent body fat.

The skinfold thickness test is performed with the aid of pressure calipers* (see Figure 2.17), and several sites must be measured to reflect the total percentage of fat: triceps, suprailium, and thigh skinfolds for women; and chest, abdomen, and thigh for men. All measurements should be taken on the right side of the body with the subject standing.

*An inexpensive, yet reliable skinfold caliper can be obtained from Fat Control, Inc., P.O. Box 10117, Towson, MD 21204, (301) 296-1993.

FIGURE 2.17

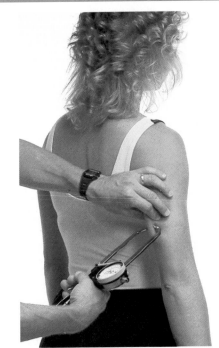

Skinfold thickness technique for body composition assessment.

The correct anatomical landmarks for skinfolds are (see Figure 2.18):

Chest: a diagonal fold halfway between the shoulder crease and the nipple.

Abdomen: a vertical fold about one inch to the right of the umbilicus.

Triceps: a vertical fold on the back of the upper arm, halfway between the shoulder and the arm.

Thigh: a vertical fold on the front of the thigh, midway between the knee and the hip.

Suprailium: a diagonal fold above the crest of the ilium (on the side of the hip).

FIGURE 2.18

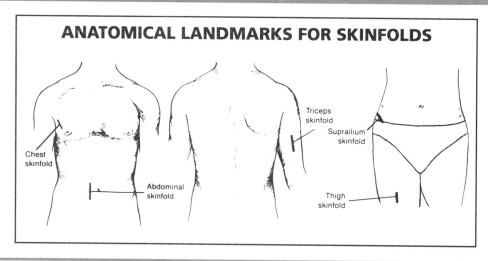

ANATOMICAL LANDMARKS FOR SKINFOLDS

Chest skinfold

Abdominal skinfold

Triceps skinfold

Suprailium skinfold

Thigh skinfold

Each site is measured by grasping a double thickness of skin firmly with the thumb and forefinger, pulling the fold slightly away from the muscle tissue. Hold the calipers perpendicular to the fold, and take the measurements one-half inch below the finger hold. Measure each site three times and read the values to the nearest .1 to .5 mm. Record the average of the two closest readings as the final value. Take the readings without delay to avoid excessive compression of the skinfold. Releasing and refolding the skinfold is required between readings. Be sure to wear shorts, a loose fitting t-shirt (no leotards), and do not use lotion on your skin the day when skinfolds are to be determined.

After determining the average value for each site, percent fat can be obtained by adding together all three skinfold measurements and looking up the respective values in Tables 2.7 for women, 2.8 for men under 40, and Table 2.9 for men over 40. Then proceed to compute your recommended body weight using the recommended percent body fat range given in Table 2.10 and the computation form in Figure 2.19.

The recommended percent body fat values given in Table 2.10 include essential fat and storage fat, previously discussed. For example, the recommended body fat range for women under age 30 is 17 to 25%. This indicates that only 5 to 13% of the total recommended fat is storage fat, and the other 12% is essential fat. The recommended range has been selected based on research indicating that some storage fat is required for optimal health and greater longevity.

The recommended body fat range selected in this book incorporates the recommendations of most health and fitness experts throughout the United States. If you desire to have just one target weight, you may select your body weight according to your personal preference, as long as it falls within the recommended range. The lower end of the range constitutes the physical fitness standard, the high end represents the health fitness standard.

TABLE 2.7

Percent fat estimates for women calculated from triceps, suprailium, and thigh skinfold thickness.

Sum of 3 Skinfolds	Under 22	23 to 27	28 to 32	33 to 37	38 to 42	43 to 47	48 to 52	53 to 57	Over 58
23- 25	9.7	9.9	10.2	10.4	10.7	10.9	11.2	11.4	11.7
26- 28	11.0	11.2	11.5	11.7	12.0	12.3	12.5	12.7	13.0
29- 31	12.3	12.5	12.8	13.0	13.3	13.5	13.8	14.0	14.3
32- 34	13.6	13.8	14.0	14.3	14.5	14.8	15.0	15.3	15.5
35- 37	14.8	15.0	15.3	15.5	15.8	16.0	16.3	16.5	16.8
38- 40	16.0	16.3	16.5	16.7	17.0	17.2	17.5	17.7	18.0
41- 43	17.2	17.4	17.7	17.9	18.2	18.4	18.7	18.9	19.2
44- 46	18.3	18.6	18.8	19.1	19.3	19.6	19.8	20.1	20.3
47- 49	19.5	19.7	20.0	20.2	20.5	20.7	21.0	21.2	21.5
50- 52	20.6	20.8	21.1	21.3	21.6	21.8	22.1	22.3	22.6
53- 55	21.7	21.9	22.1	22.4	22.6	22.9	23.1	23.4	23.6
56- 58	22.7	23.0	23.2	23.4	23.7	23.9	24.2	24.4	24.7
59- 61	23.7	24.0	24.2	24.5	24.7	25.0	25.2	25.5	25.7
62- 64	24.7	25.0	25.2	25.5	25.7	26.0	26.2	26.4	26.7
65- 67	25.7	25.9	26.2	26.4	26.7	26.9	27.2	27.4	27.7
68- 70	26.6	26.9	27.1	27.4	27.6	27.9	28.1	28.4	28.6
71- 73	27.5	27.8	28.0	28.3	28.5	28.8	29.0	29.3	29.5
74- 76	28.4	28.7	28.9	29.2	29.4	29.7	29.9	30.2	30.4
77- 79	29.3	29.5	29.8	30.0	30.3	30.5	30.8	31.0	31.3
80- 82	30.1	30.4	30.6	30.9	31.1	31.4	31.6	31.9	32.1
83- 85	30.9	31.2	31.4	31.7	31.9	32.2	32.4	32.7	32.9
86- 88	31.7	32.0	32.2	32.5	32.7	32.9	33.2	33.4	33.7
89- 91	32.5	32.7	33.0	33.2	33.5	33.7	33.9	34.2	34.4
92- 94	33.2	33.4	33.7	33.9	34.2	34.4	34.7	34.9	35.2
95- 97	33.9	34.1	34.4	34.6	34.9	35.1	35.4	35.6	35.9
98-100	34.6	34.8	35.1	35.3	35.5	35.8	36.0	36.3	36.5
101-103	35.2	35.4	35.7	35.9	36.2	36.4	36.7	36.9	37.2
104-106	35.8	36.1	36.3	36.6	36.8	37.1	37.3	37.5	37.8
107-109	36.4	36.7	36.9	37.1	37.4	37.6	37.9	38.1	38.4
110-112	37.0	37.2	37.5	37.7	38.0	38.2	38.5	38.7	38.9
113-115	37.5	37.8	38.0	38.2	38.5	38.7	39.0	39.2	39.5
116-118	38.0	38.3	38.5	38.8	39.0	39.3	39.5	39.7	40.0
119-121	38.5	38.7	39.0	39.2	39.5	39.7	40.0	40.2	40.5
122-124	39.0	39.2	39.4	39.7	39.9	40.2	40.4	40.7	40.9
125-127	39.4	39.6	39.9	40.1	40.4	40.6	40.9	41.1	41.4
128-130	39.8	40.0	40.3	40.5	40.8	41.0	41.3	41.5	41.8

Body density calculated based on the generalized equation for predicting body density of women developed by Jackson, A. S., M. L. Pollock. *British Journal of Nutrition* 40:497-504, 1978. Percent body fat determined from the calculated body density using the Siri formula (W. E. Siri, *Body Composition from Fluid Spaces and Density*, Berkeley, CA; University of California, Donner Laboratory of Medical Physics, 1956).

Fitness and Wellness

TABLE 2.8

Percent fat estimates for men under 40 calculated from chest, abdomen, and thigh skinfold thickness.

Sum of 3 Skinfolds	Under 19	20 to 22	23 to 25	26 to 28	29 to 31	32 to 34	35 to 37	38 to 40
8- 10	.9	1.3	1.6	2.0	2.3	2.7	3.0	3.3
11- 13	1.9	2.3	2.6	3.0	3.3	3.7	4.0	4.3
14- 16	2.9	3.3	3.6	3.9	4.3	4.6	5.0	5.3
17- 19	3.9	4.2	4.6	4.9	5.3	5.6	6.0	6.3
20- 22	4.8	5.2	5.5	5.9	6.2	6.6	6.9	7.3
23- 25	5.8	6.2	6.5	6.8	7.2	7.5	7.9	8.2
26- 28	6.8	7.1	7.5	7.8	8.1	8.5	8.8	9.2
29- 31	7.7	8.0	8.4	8.7	9.1	9.4	9.8	10.1
32- 34	8.6	9.0	9.3	9.7	10.0	10.4	10.7	11.1
35- 37	9.5	9.9	10.2	10.6	10.9	11.3	11.6	12.0
38- 40	10.5	10.8	11.2	11.5	11.8	12.2	12.5	12.9
41- 43	11.4	11.7	12.1	12.4	12.7	13.1	13.4	13.8
44- 46	12.2	12.6	12.9	13.3	13.6	14.0	14.3	14.7
47- 49	13.1	13.5	13.8	14.2	14.5	14.9	15.2	15.5
50- 52	14.0	14.3	14.7	15.0	15.4	15.7	16.1	16.4
53- 55	14.8	15.2	15.5	15.9	16.2	16.6	16.9	17.3
56- 58	15.7	16.0	16.4	16.7	17.1	17.4	17.8	18.1
59- 61	16.5	16.9	17.2	17.6	17.9	18.3	18.6	19.0
62- 64	17.4	17.7	18.1	18.4	18.8	19.1	19.4	19.8
65- 67	18.2	18.5	18.9	19.2	19.6	19.9	20.3	20.6
68- 70	19.0	19.3	19.7	20.0	20.4	20.7	21.1	21.4
71- 73	19.8	20.1	20.5	20.8	21.2	21.5	21.9	22.2
74- 76	20.6	20.9	21.3	21.6	22.0	22.2	22.7	23.0
77- 79	21.4	21.7	22.1	22.4	22.8	23.1	23.4	23.8
80- 82	22.1	22.5	22.8	23.2	23.5	23.9	24.2	24.6
83- 85	22.9	23.2	23.6	23.9	24.3	24.6	25.0	25.3
86- 88	23.6	24.0	24.3	24.7	25.0	25.4	25.7	26.1
89- 91	24.4	24.7	25.1	25.4	25.8	26.1	26.5	26.8
92- 94	25.1	25.5	25.8	26.2	26.5	26.9	27.2	27.5
95- 97	25.8	26.2	26.5	26.9	27.2	27.6	27.9	28.3
98-100	26.6	26.9	27.3	27.6	27.9	28.3	28.6	29.0
101-103	27.3	27.6	28.0	28.3	28.6	29.0	29.3	29.7
104-106	27.9	28.3	28.6	29.0	29.3	29.7	30.0	30.4
107-109	28.6	29.0	29.3	29.7	30.0	30.4	30.7	31.1
110-112	29.3	29.6	30.0	30.3	30.7	31.0	31.4	31.7
113-115	30.0	30.3	30.7	31.0	31.3	31.7	32.0	32.4
116-118	30.6	31.0	31.3	31.6	32.0	32.3	32.7	33.0
119-121	31.3	31.6	32.0	32.3	32.6	33.0	33.3	33.7
122-124	31.9	32.2	32.6	32.9	33.3	33.6	34.0	34.3
125-127	32.5	32.9	33.2	33.5	33.9	34.2	34.6	34.9
128-130	33.1	33.5	33.8	34.2	34.5	34.9	35.2	35.5

Body density calculated based on the generalized equation for predicting body density of men developed by Jackson, A.S., and M. L. Pollock. *British Journal of Nutrition* 40:497-504, 1978. Percent body fat determined from the calculated body density using the Siri formula (W. E. Siri, *Body Composition from Fluid Spaces and Density*, Berkeley, CA; University of California, Donner Laboratory of Medical Physics, 1956).

Physical Fitness Assessment

TABLE 2.9

Percent fat estimates for men over 40 calculated from chest, abdomen, and thigh skinfold thickness.

Sum of 3 Skinfolds	Age to the Last Year							
	41 to 43	44 to 46	47 to 49	50 to 52	53 to 55	56 to 58	59 to 61	Over 62
8- 10	3.7	4.0	4.4	4.7	5.1	5.4	5.8	6.1
11- 13	4.7	5.0	5.4	5.7	6.1	6.4	6.8	7.1
14- 16	5.7	6.0	6.4	6.7	7.1	7.4	7.8	8.1
17- 19	6.7	7.0	7.4	7.7	8.1	8.4	8.7	9.1
20- 22	7.6	8.0	8.3	8.7	9.0	9.4	9.7	10.1
23- 25	8.6	8.9	9.3	9.6	10.0	10.3	10.7	11.0
26- 28	9.5	9.9	10.2	10.6	10.9	11.3	11.6	12.0
29- 31	10.5	10.8	11.2	11.5	11.9	12.2	12.6	12.9
32- 34	11.4	11.8	12.1	12.4	12.8	13.1	13.5	13.8
35- 37	12.3	12.7	13.0	13.4	13.7	14.1	14.4	14.8
38- 40	13.2	13.6	13.9	14.3	14.6	15.0	15.3	15.7
41- 43	14.1	14.5	14.8	15.2	15.5	15.9	16.2	16.6
44- 46	15.0	15.4	15.7	16.1	16.4	16.8	17.1	17.5
47- 49	15.9	16.2	16.6	16.9	17.3	17.6	18.0	18.3
50- 52	16.8	17.1	17.5	17.8	18.2	18.5	18.8	19.2
53- 55	17.6	18.0	18.3	18.7	19.0	19.4	19.7	20.1
56- 58	18.5	18.8	19.2	19.5	19.9	20.2	20.6	20.9
59- 61	19.3	19.7	20.0	20.4	20.7	21.0	21.4	21.7
62- 64	20.1	20.5	20.8	21.2	21.5	21.9	22.2	22.6
65- 67	21.0	21.3	21.7	22.0	22.4	22.7	23.0	23.4
68- 70	21.8	22.1	22.5	22.8	23.2	23.5	23.9	24.2
71- 73	22.6	22.9	23.3	23.6	24.0	24.3	24.7	25.0
74- 76	23.4	23.7	24.1	24.4	24.8	25.1	25.4	25.8
77- 79	24.1	24.5	24.8	25.2	25.5	25.9	26.2	26.6
80- 82	24.9	25.3	25.6	26.0	26.3	26.6	27.0	27.3
83- 85	25.7	26.0	26.4	26.7	27.1	27.4	27.8	28.1
86- 88	26.4	26.8	27.1	27.5	27.8	28.2	28.5	28.9
89- 91	27.2	27.5	27.9	38.2	28.6	28.9	29.2	29.6
92- 94	27.9	28.2	28.6	28.9	29.3	29.6	30.0	30.3
95- 97	28.6	29.0	29.3	29.7	30.0	30.4	30.7	31.1
98-100	29.3	29.7	30.0	30.4	30.7	31.1	31.4	31.8
101-103	30.0	30.4	30.7	31.1	31.4	31.8	32.1	32.5
104-106	30.7	31.1	31.4	31.8	32.1	32.5	32.8	33.2
107-109	31.4	31.8	32.1	32.4	32.8	33.1	33.5	33.8
110-112	32.1	32.4	32.8	33.1	33.5	33.8	34.2	34.5
113-115	32.7	33.1	33.4	33.8	34.1	34.5	34.8	35.2
116-118	33.4	33.7	34.1	34.4	34.8	35.1	35.5	35.8
119-121	34.0	34.4	34.7	35.1	35.4	35.8	36.1	36.5
122-124	34.7	35.0	35.4	35.7	36.1	36.4	36.7	37.1
125-127	35.3	35.6	36.0	36.3	36.7	37.0	37.4	37.7
128-130	35.9	36.2	36.6	36.9	37.3	37.6	38.0	38.5

Body density calculated based on the generalized equation for predicting body density of men developed by Jackson, A. S., and M. L. Pollock. *British Journal of Nutrition* 40:497-504, 1978. Percent body fat determined from the calculated body density using the Siri formula (W. E. Siri, *Body Composition from Fluid Spaces and Density*, Berkeley, CA: University of California, Donner Laboratory of Medical Physics, 1956).

TABLE 2.10

Recommended Body Composition According to Percent Body Fat

Age	Males	Females
≤29	12–20%	17–25%
30–49	13–21%	18–26%
≥50	14–22%	19–27%

▢ High physical fitness standard

▉ Health fitness standard

Waist-to-Hip Ratio

Recent scientific evidence also suggests that the way people store fat may also affect the risk for disease. Some individuals have a tendency to store high amounts of fat in the abdominal area, while others store it primarily around the hips and thighs (gluteal femoral fat).

Data indicates that obese individuals with high abdominal fat are clearly at higher risk for coronary heart disease, congestive heart failure, hypertension, strokes, and diabetes than obese people with similar amounts of total body fat, but stored primarily in the hips and

FIGURE 2.19

Recommended Body Weight Determination

A.   Current Body Weight (BW): _____ lbs

B.   Current Percent Fat (%F): _____ %

C.   Fat Weight (FW) = BW × %F* = _____ × _____ = _____ lbs

D.   Lean Body Mass (LBM) = BW – FW = _____ – _____ = _____ lbs

E.   Age: _____

F.   Recommended Fat Percent (RFP) Range (see Table 2.10):

   Low End of Recommended Fat Percent Range (LRFP): _____ % (Physical Fitness Standard)

   High End of Recommended Fat Percent Range (HRFP): _____ % (Health Fitness Standard)

G.   Recommended Body Weight Range

   Low End of Recommended Body Weight Range (LRBW) = LBM/(1.0 – LRFP*)

   LRBW = _____ / (1.0 – _____) = _____ lbs

   High End of Recommended Body Weight Range (HRBW) = LBM/(1.0 – HRFP*)

   HRBW = _____ / (1.0 – _____) = _____ lbs

   Recommended Body Weight Range: _____ to _____ lbs

*Express percentages in decimal form (e.g., 25% = .25)

thighs. Relatively new evidence also indicates that among individuals with high abdominal fat, those whose fat deposits are around internal organs (visceral fat) are at even greater risk for disease than those whose abdominal fat is primarily beneath the skin (sub-cutaneous fat).

Because of the increased risk for disease in individuals who tend to store high amounts of fat in the abdominal area, as opposed to the hips and thighs, a waist-to-hip ratio test was recently designed by a panel of scientists appointed by the National Academy of Sciences and the Dietary Guidelines Advisory Council for the U.S. Departments of Agriculture and Health and Human Services. The panel recommends that men need to lose weight if the waist-to-hip ratio is 1.0 or higher. Women need to lose weight if the ratio is .85 or higher. The waist-to-hip ratio for a man with a 40-inch waist and a 38-inch hip would be 1.05 (40 ÷ 38). Such a ratio may be indicative of increased risk for disease. Using a simple tape measure, you may determine your own waist-to-hip ratio and the results can be recorded in Figure 2.20.

Effects of Exercise and Diet on Body Composition

If you engage in a diet/exercise program, you should repeat body composition measurements about once a month to monitor changes in lean and fat tissue. This is important because lean body mass is affected by weight reduction programs as well as physical activity. A negative caloric balance does lead to a decrease in lean body mass. These effects will

TABLE 2.20
Waist-to-Hip Ratio Computation Form

Waist (inches): _____

Hip (inches) _____

Ratio (waist/hip) _____

Recommended Standard

Men: <1.0

Women: <.85

be explained in more detail in Chapter 5. As lean body mass changes, so will your recommended body weight.

Changes in body composition resulting from a weight control/exercise program was illustrated by a co-ed aerobics course taught during a 6-week summer term. Students participated in aerobic dance routines four times a week, 60 minutes each time. On the first and the last day of class several physiological parameters, including body composition, were assessed. Students also were given information on diet and nutrition and basically followed their own weight control program. At the end of the 6 weeks, the average weight loss for the entire class was only 3 pounds. When body composition was assessed, however, class members were surprised to find out that the average fat loss was actually 6 pounds, accompanied by a 3-pound increase in lean body mass (see Figure 2.21).

FIGURE 2.21

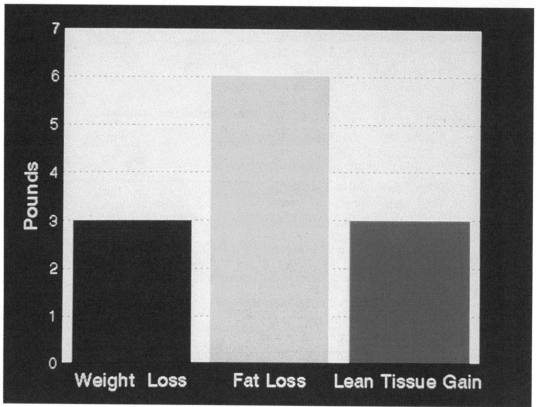

Effects of a six-week aerobics exercise program on body composition.

Research conducted at The University of Texas of the Permian Basin, Odessa, TX, 1985.

Exercise Prescription

3

KEY CONCEPTS

- Exercise readiness
- Cardiovascular endurance
- Aerobic exercise
- Cardiovascular training zone
- Muscular strength
- Muscular endurance
- Overload principle
- Specificity of training
- Isometric exercise
- Isotonic exercise
- Isokinetic exercise
- Muscular flexibility
- Slow-sustained stretching
- Proprioceptive neuromuscular facilitation
- Exercise adherence

OBJECTIVES

- Learn to write personalized cardiovascular, strength, and flexibility exercise programs.
- Be able to write fitness goals.
- Learn basic skills to enhance exercise adherence.

A most inspiring story illustrating what fitness can do for a person's health and well-being is that of George Snell from Sandy, Utah. At age 45, Snell weighed approximately 400 pounds, his blood pressure was 220/180, he was blind because of diabetes he did not know he had, and his blood glucose level was 487. Snell determined to do something about his physical and medical condition, so he started a walking/jogging program. After about 8 months of conditioning, he had lost almost 200 pounds, his eyesight had returned, his glucose level was down to 67, and he was taken off medication. Two months later, less than 10 months after initiating his personal exercise program, he completed his first marathon, a running course of 26.2 miles!

Research results have established that participating in a lifetime exercise program greatly contributes to good health. Nonetheless, too many individuals who exercise regularly are surprised to find, when they take a battery of fitness tests, that they may not be as conditioned as they thought they were. Although these individuals may be exercising regularly, they most likely are not following the basic principles of exercise prescription; therefore, they do not reap significant benefits.

All programs must be individualized to obtain optimal results. Our bodies are not all alike, and fitness levels and needs vary among individuals. The information presented in this chapter provides you with the necessary guidelines to write a personalized cardiovascular, strength, and flexibility exercise program to promote and maintain physical fitness and wellness. Information on weight control to achieve recommended body composition (the fourth component of physical fitness), is given in Chapter 5.

EXERCISE READINESS

Surveys indicate that less than 20% of the adult population in the United States exercises vigorously enough to develop the cardiovascular system. Furthermore, more than half of the people who start exercising drop out during the first 6 months of the program. Sports psychologists are trying to find out why some people habitually exercise and many do not. All of the benefits of exercise cannot help unless people commit to a lifetime program of physical activity.

Are you willing to give exercise a try? The first step is to decide positively that you will try. To help you make this decision, start with Figure 3.1. Make a list of the advantages and disadvantages of incorporating exercise into your lifestyle. Your list may include things such as: It will make me feel better. I will lose weight. I will have more energy. It will lower risk for chronic diseases. Your list of disadvantages may include: I don't want to take the time. I'm too out of shape. There's no good place to exercise. I don't have the willpower to do it. When the reasons for exercise outweigh the reasons for not exercising, it will become easier to try. A second questionnaire that may provide answers about your readiness to start an exercise program is provided in Figure 3.2. Carefully read each statement and circle the number that best describes your feelings. Be completely honest in your answers. You are evaluated in four categories: mastery (self-control), attitude, health, and commitment. The higher you score in any category — mastery, for example — the more important that reason is for you to exercise.

Scores can vary from 4 to 16. A score of 12 and above is a strong indicator that that factor is important to you, whereas 8 and below is low. If you score 12 or more points in each category, your chances of initiating and sticking to an exercise program are good. If you do not score at least 12 points in three categories, your chances of succeeding at exercise may be slim. You need to be better informed about the benefits of exercise, and a retraining process may be helpful. More tips on how to enhance commitment to exercise are provided later in the chapter.

FIGURE 3.1

Advantages and disadvantages of adding exercise to your lifestyle.

Name:_____Date: _____

Advantages of starting an exercise program

1. _____

2. _____

3. _____

4. _____

5. _____

6. _____

7. _____

8. _____

Disadvantages of starting an exercise program

1. _____

2. _____

3. _____

4. _____

5. _____

6. _____

7. _____

8. _____

FIGURE 3.2

Exercise Readiness Questionnaire

Name:_____   Date: _____

Carefully read each statement and circle the number that best describes your feelings in each statement. Please be completely honest with your answers.

	Strongly Agree	Mildly Agree	Mildly Disagree	Strongly Disagree
1. I can walk, ride a bike (or a wheelchair), swim, or walk in a shallow pool.	4	3	2	1
2. I enjoy exercise.	4	3	2	1
3. I believe exercise can help decrease the risk for disease and premature mortality.	4	3	2	1
4. I believe exercise contributes to better health.	4	3	2	1
5. I have previously participated in an exercise program.	4	3	2	1
6. I have experienced the feeling of being physically fit.	4	3	2	1
7. I can envision myself exercising.	4	3	2	1
8. I am contemplating an exercise program.	4	3	2	1
9. I am willing to stop contemplating and give exercise a try for a few weeks.	4	3	2	1
10. I am willing to set aside time at least three times a week for exercise.	4	3	2	1
11. I can find a place to exercise (the streets, a park, a YMCA, a health club).	4	3	2	1
12. I can find other people who would like to exercise with me.	4	3	2	1
13. I will exercise when I am moody, fatigued, and even when the weather is bad.	4	3	2	1
14. I am willing to spend a small amount of money for adequate exercise clothing (shoes, shorts, leotards, or swimsuit).	4	3	2	1
15. If I have any doubts about my present state of health, I will see a physician before beginning an exercise program.	4	3	2	1
16. Exercise will make me feel better and improve my quality of life.	4	3	2	1

Scoring Your Test:

This questionnaire allows you to examine your readiness for exercise. You have been evaluated in four categories: mastery (self-control), attitude, health, and commitment. Mastery indicates that you can be in control of your exercise program. Attitude examines your mental disposition toward exercise. Health provides evidence of the wellness benefits of exercise. Commitment shows dedication and resolution to carry out the exercise program. Write the number you circled after each statement in the corresponding spaces below. Add the scores on each line to get your totals. Scores can vary from 4 to 16. A score of 12 and above is a strong indicator that that factor is important to you, and 8 and below is low. If you score 12 or more points in each category, your chances of initiating and adhering to an exercise program are good. If you fail to score at least 12 points in three categories, your chances of succeeding at exercise may be slim. You need to be better informed about the benefits of exercise, and a retraining process may be required.

Mastery:	1._____	+ 5._____	+ 6._____	+ 9._____	= _____
Attitude:	2._____	+ 7._____	+ 8._____	+ 13._____	= _____
Health:	3._____	+ 4._____	+ 15._____	+ 16._____	= _____
Commitment:	10._____	+ 11._____	+ 12._____	+ 14._____	= _____

CARDIOVASCULAR ENDURANCE

A sound cardiovascular endurance program greatly contributes to enhancing and maintaining good health. Although physical fitness has four components, cardiovascular endurance (see Figure 3.3) is the single most important one. Even though certain amounts of muscular strength and flexibility are necessary in normal daily activities, a person can get away without having a lot of strength and flexibility but cannot do without a good cardiovascular system.

FIGURE 3.3

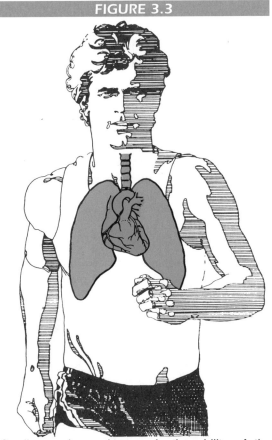

Cardiovascular endurance is the ability of the heart, lungs, and blood vessels to deliver adequate amounts of oxygen to the cells to meet the demands of prolonged physical activity.

Principles of Cardiovascular Exercise Prescription

The objective of aerobic training is to improve the capacity of the cardiovascular system. To accomplish this, the heart muscle has to be overloaded like any other muscle in the human body. Just as the biceps muscle in the upper arm is developed through strength training, the heart muscle has to be exercised to increase in size, strength, and efficiency. To better understand how the cardiovascular system can be developed, we have to be familiar with the four basic principles of intensity, mode, duration, and frequency of exercise.

The American College of Sports Medicine (ACSM) recommends that a medical exam and a diagnostic exercise stress test (see Figure 2.2, Chapter 2) be administered prior to vigorous exercise by apparently healthy men over age 40 and women over 50. ACSM has defined "vigorous exercise" as an exercise intensity that provides a "substantial challenge" to the participant or one that cannot be maintained for 20 continuous minutes.

Intensity of Exercise

Intensity refers to how hard a person has to exercise to improve cardiovascular endurance. Muscles have to be overloaded for them to develop. While the training stimulus to develop the biceps muscle can be accomplished with curl-up exercises, the stimulus for the cardiovascular system is provided by making the heart pump at a higher rate for a certain period of time.

Cardiovascular development occurs when the heart is working between 50 and 85% of heart rate reserve. Development is accelerated when the heart is working closer to 85% of heart rate reserve. For this reason, many experts prescribe exercise between 70 and 85% for young people. Exercise intensity can be easily calculated and training can be monitored by checking your pulse. To determine the intensity of exercise or cardiovascular training zone, follow these steps:

1. Estimate your maximal heart rate (MHR) according to the following formula:

   MHR = 220 minus age (220 − age)

2. Check your resting heart rate (RHR) some time after you have been sitting quietly for 15 to 20 minutes. You may take your pulse for 30 seconds and multiply by 2, or take it for a full minute. As explained in Chapter 2, you can check your pulse on the wrist by placing two or three fingers over the radial artery or over the carotid artery in the neck (see Figures 2.3 and 2.4).

3. Determine the heart rate reserve (HRR) by subtracting the resting heart rate from the maximal heart rate (HRR = MHR − RHR).

4. Calculate the training intensities (TI) at 50%, 70%, and 85%. Multiply the heart rate reserve by the respective 50, 70, and 85 percentages, and then add the resting heart rate to both of these figures (for example, 85% TI = HRR × .85 + RHR).

   Example. The 50, 70, and 85 percent training intensities for a 20-year-old with a resting heart rate of 68 beats per minute (bpm) would be:

   MHR: 220 − 20 = 200 bpm

   RHR = 68 bpm

   HRR: 200 − 68 = 132 beats

   50% TI = (132 × .50) + 68 = 134 bpm

   70% TI = (132 × .70) + 68 = 160 bpm

   85% TI = (132 × .85) + 68 = 180 bpm

   Cardiovascular training
      zone: 134 to 180 bpm

The cardiovascular training zone indicates that whenever you exercise to improve the cardiovascular system, you should maintain the heart rate between the 50 and 85% training intensities to obtain adequate development. If you have been physically inactive, you should train around the 50% intensity during the first 4 to 6 weeks of the exercise program. After the first few weeks, you should exercise between 70 and 85% training intensity.

Following a few weeks of training, you may have a considerably lower resting heart rate (10 to 20 beats in 8 to 12 weeks). Therefore, you should recompute your target zone periodically. You can compute your own cardiovascular training zone by using the form in Figure 3.4. Once you have reached an ideal level of cardiovascular endurance, training in the 50 to 85% range will allow you to maintain your fitness level.

To develop the cardiovascular system, you do not have to exercise above the 85% rate. From a fitness standpoint, training above this percentage will not give extra benefits and may actually be unsafe for some individuals. For unconditioned people and older adults, cardiovascular training should be conducted around the 50% rate to discourage potential problems associated with high-intensity exercise.

Mode of Exercise

The type of exercise that develops the cardiovascular system has to be aerobic in nature. Once you have established your cardiovascular training zone, *any activity or combination of activities that will get your heart rate up to the training zone and keep it there for as long as you exercise will provide adequate development.* Examples of these activities are walking, jogging, aerobics, swimming, water aerobics, cross-country skiing, rope skipping, cycling, racquetball, stair climbing, and stationary running or cycling.

Duration of Exercise

The general recommendation is that a person *train between 20 and 60 minutes per session.* The duration is based on how intensely

FIGURE 3.4

Cardiovascular Exercise Prescription Form

Intensity of Exercise

1. Estimate your own maximal heart rate (MHR)

   MHR = 220 minus age (220 – age)

   MHR = _____ – _____ = _____ bpm

2. Resting Heart Rate (RHR) = _____ bpm

3. Heart Rate Reserve (HRR) = MHR – RHR

   HRR = _____ – _____ = _____ beats

4. Training Intensity (TI) = HRR × %TI + RHR

   50% TI = _____ × .50 + _____ = _____ bpm

   70% TI = _____ × .70 + _____ = _____ bpm

   85% TI = _____ × .85 + _____ = _____ bpm

5. Cardiovascular Training Zone. The optimum cardiovascular training zone is found between the 70 and 85% training intensities. Individuals who have been physically inactive or are in the poor or fair cardiovascular fitness categories, however, should follow a 50% training intensity during the first few weeks of the exercise program.

   Cardiovascular Training Zone: _____ (70% TI) to _____ (85% TI)

Mode of Exercise: List any activity or combination of aerobic activities that you will use in your cardiovascular training program:

_____

Duration of Exercise: Indicate the length of your exercise sessions: _____ minutes

Frequency of Exercise: Indicate the days you will exercise:

_____

Student's Name: _____ Date: _____

Signature: _____

a person trains. If the training is done around 85%, 20 minutes are sufficient. At 50% intensity, the person should train for at least 30 minutes. As mentioned under "intensity of exercise," unconditioned people and older adults should train at lower percentages; therefore, the activity should be carried out over a longer time.

If individuals are on a weight loss program, 45- to 60-minute exercise sessions of low to moderate intensity, conducted five or six days per week, are recommended. Longer exercise sessions increase caloric expenditure for faster weight reduction (see Chapter 5).

Frequency of Exercise

Ideally, a person should *engage in aerobic exercise three to five times per week.* When starting an exercise program, three to five 20- to 30-minute training sessions per week improve maximal oxygen uptake. Further improvements are minimal when training is conducted more than five days per week. Three 20- to 30-minute training sessions per week, on non-consecutive days, will maintain cardiovascular fitness as long as the heart rate is in the appropriate target zone. A summary of the cardiovascular exercise prescription guidelines, according to the ACSM, is provided in Figure 3.5.

FIGURE 3.5

Cardiovascular Exercise Prescription Guidelines*

Activity:	Aerobic (examples: walking, jogging, cycling, swimming, aerobics, racquetball, soccer, stair climbing)
Intensity:	50-85% of heart rate reserve
Duration:	20-60 minutes of continuous aerobic activity
Frequency:	3 to 5 days per week

*Source: "The Recommended Quantity and Quality of Exercise for Developing and Maintaining Cardiorespiratory and Muscular Fitness in Healthy Adults by the American College of Sports Medicine," Med. Sci. Sports Exerc. 22:265-274, 1990.

MUSCULAR STRENGTH AND ENDURANCE

The capacity of muscle cells to exert force increases and decreases according to demands placed upon the muscular system. If specific muscle cells are overloaded beyond their normal use, such as in strength training programs, the cells increase in size (hypertrophy), strength, or endurance, or some combination of these. If the demands on the muscle cells decrease, such as in sedentary living or required rest because of illness or injury, the cells decrease in size (atrophy) and lose strength.

Overload Principle

The overload principle states that for strength or endurance to improve, the demands placed on the muscle must be systematically and progressively increased over time, and the resistance (weight lifted) must be of a magnitude significant enough to cause physiologic adaptation. In simpler terms, just like all other organs and systems of the human body, muscles have to be taxed beyond their regular accustomed loads to increase in physical capacity.

Specificity of Training

Muscular strength is defined as the ability to exert maximum force against resistance. Muscular endurance (also referred to as localized muscular endurance) is the ability of a muscle to exert submaximal force repeatedly over a period of time.

The principle of specificity states that for a muscle to increase in strength or endurance, the training program must be specific to obtain the desired effects. As discussed later in this section, a person attempting to increase muscular strength needs a program of few repetitions and near maximum resistance. To increase muscular endurance, the strength training program consists primarily of many repetitions at a lower resistance.

In like manner, to increase isometric (static) versus isotonic (dynamic) strength — see mode of training below — an individual must use the corresponding static or dynamic training procedures to achieve the appropriate results. If a person is trying to improve a specific movement or skill through strength increases, the selected strength-training exercises must resemble the actual movement or skill as closely as possible.

Principles of Strength-Training Prescription

Similar to the prescription of cardiovascular exercise, several principles have to be observed to improve muscular strength and endurance. These principles relate to mode, resistance, sets, and frequency of training.

Mode of Training

Two basic training methods are used to improve strength: isometric (static) and isotonic (dynamic). In isometric training, a muscle contraction produces little or no movement, such as pushing or pulling without movement against immovable objects (see Figure 3.6). In isotonic training, a muscle contraction is accompanied by movement (see Figure 3.7), such as lifting an object over the head.

Isometric training does not require much equipment. It was commonly used several years ago, but its popularity has waned. Because strength gains with isometric training are specific to the angle of muscle contraction, this type of training is beneficial in a sport such as gymnastics, which requires regular static contractions during routines.

Isotonic training can be conducted without weights, with free weights (barbells and

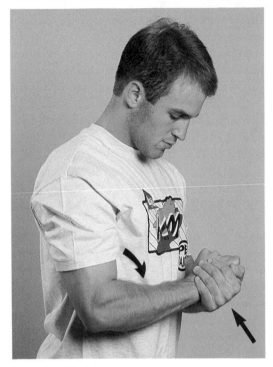

FIGURE 3.6

Isometric Training

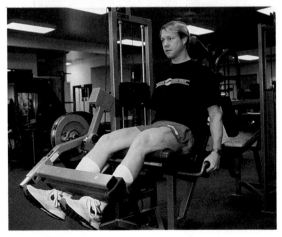

FIGURE 3.7

Isotonic Training

dumbbells), fixed resistance machines, variable resistance machines, and isokinetic equipment. When performing isotonic exercises without weights (for example, pull-ups, push-ups), with free weights, or with fixed resistance machines, a constant resistance (weight) is moved through a joint's full range of motion. The greatest resistance that can be lifted equals the maximum weight that can be moved at the weakest angle of the joint. This is due to changes in muscle length and angle of pull as the joint moves through its range of motion.

As strength training became more popular, new strength-training machines were developed. This technology brought about isokinetic and variable resistance training. These training programs require special machines equipped with mechanical devices that provide differing amounts of resistance, with the intent of overloading the muscle group maximally through the entire range of motion. A distinction of *isokinetic training* (see Figure 3.8) is that the speed of the muscle contraction is kept constant because the machine provides

FIGURE 3.8

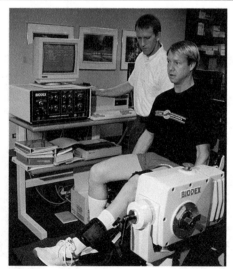

Isokinetic Training
(Courtesy of the Idaho Sports Medicine Institute, Boise, Idaho)

resistance to match the user's force through the range of motion. Because of the expense of the equipment needed for isokinetic training, this type of program is usually reserved for clinical settings (physical therapy), research laboratories, and professional sports.

The mode of training depends mainly on the type of equipment available and the specific objective of the training program. Isotonic training is the most popular mode for strength training. Its primary advantage is that strength is gained through the full range of motion. Most daily activities are isotonic. We are constantly lifting, pushing, and pulling objects, which requires strength through a complete range of motion. Another advantage is that improvements are easily measured by the amount lifted.

The benefits of isokinetic and variable resistance training are similar to those of the other isotonic training methods. Theoretically, strength gains should be better because maximum resistance is applied through the entire range of motion. Research, however, has not shown this type of training to be more effective than other modes of isotonic training. A possible advantage is that specific speeds in various sport skills can be more closely duplicated with isokinetic strength training, which may enhance performance (specificity of training). A disadvantage is that the equipment is not readily available to many people.

Resistance

Resistance in strength training is the equivalent of intensity in cardiovascular exercise prescription. The amount of resistance, or weight lifted, depends on whether the individual is trying to develop muscular strength or muscular endurance.

To stimulate strength development, a resistance of approximately 80% of the maximum capacity is recommended. For example, a person whose one repetition maximum (1 RM) for a given exercise is 150 pounds should work with at least 120 pounds (150 × .80). Using less than 80% will foster muscular endurance rather than strength. The time factor involved in constantly determining the 1 RM on each lift to ensure working above 80% is prohibitive. Therefore, a rule of thumb widely accepted by many authors and coaches is that *individuals should perform between three and ten repetitions maximum (3 to 10 RM) for adequate strength gains.*

For example, if a person is training with a resistance of 120 pounds and cannot lift it more than ten times, the training stimulus is adequate for strength development. Once the person can lift weight more than ten times, the resistance should be increased by 5 to 10 pounds and the person again should build up to 10 RM. Training with more than ten repetitions develops muscular endurance primarily. A person training with 20 maximum or near maximum repetitions, for example, will experience incremental increases in localized muscular endurance (localized to the specific muscle groups involved in the exercise).

Strength research indicates that the closer a person trains to the 1 RM, the greater are the strength gains. A disadvantage of constantly working at or near the 1 RM is that it increases the risk for injury. Highly trained athletes seeking maximum strength development do 3 to 6 RM. Working around 10 RM seems to produce the best results in terms of muscular hypertrophy.

From a health-fitness point of view, 6 to 10 RM are ideal. We live in an "isotonic world" in which muscular strength and endurance are both required to lead an enjoyable life. Therefore, working near the 10 RM threshold seems best to improve overall performance.

Sets

A set in strength training has been defined as *the number of repetitions performed for a given exercise.* For example, a person lifting 120 pounds eight times performs one set of eight repetitions (1 × 8 × 120). The number of sets recommended for optimum development is three sets per exercise.

Because of the characteristics of muscle fiber, the number of sets that can be done is limited. As the number of sets increases, so does the amount of muscle fatigue and subsequent recovery time; therefore, strength gains may be lessened by performing too many sets. *A recommended program for beginners in their first year of training is three heavy sets,* up to the maximum number of repetitions, preceded by one or two light warm-up sets using about 50% of the 1 RM.

To make the exercise program more time-effective, two or three exercises that require different muscle groups may be alternated. In this way, a person will not have to wait too long before proceeding to a new set on a different exercise. For example, bench press, leg extensions, and sit-ups may be combined so the person can go almost directly from one set to the next.

To avoid muscle soreness and stiffness, new participants ought to build up gradually to the three sets of maximal repetitions. This can be done by doing only one set of each exercise with a lighter resistance on the first day. During the second session, two sets of each exercise can be done, one light and the second with the regular resistance. During the third session, three sets could be performed, one light and two heavy ones. After that, a person should be able to do all three heavy sets.

Frequency of Training

Strength training should be done either with *a total body workout three times per week,* or more frequently if using a split-body routine (upper body one day and lower body the next). After a maximum strength workout, the muscles should be rested for about 48 hours to allow adequate recovery. If not completely recovered in two or three days, the person is most likely overtraining and therefore not reaping the full benefits of the program. In that case, a decrease in the total number of sets or exercises, or both, performed during the previous workout is recommended.

To achieve significant strength gains, a minimum of eight weeks of consecutive training is needed. Once an ideal level of strength is achieved, one training session per week will be sufficient to maintain the new strength level.

Designing Your Own Strength-Training Program

Two strength-training programs, presented in Appendix B, have been developed to provide a complete body workout. Only a minimum of equipment is required for the first program "Strength-Training Exercises Without Weights" (Exercises 1 through 10). This program can be conducted within the walls of your own home. Your body weight is used as the primary resistance for most exercises. A few exercises call for a friend's help or basic implements from around your house to provide greater resistance. The second program, "Strength-Training Exercises With Weights" (exercises 11 through 17), require machines such as those shown in the various photographs. Many of these exercises can also be performed with free weights.

Depending on the facilities available to you, choose one of the two training programs outlined in Appendix B. The resistance and the number of repetitions that you use should be based on whether you want to increase muscular strength or muscular endurance. Do up to ten RM for strength gains, and more than ten for muscular endurance. As pointed out, three training sessions per week on nonconsecutive days is an ideal arrangement for proper development. Since both strength and endurance are required in daily activities, three sets of about ten RM for each exercise are enough. In doing this, you will obtain good strength gains and yet be close to the endurance threshold.

Perhaps the only exercise that calls for more than ten repetitions is the abdominal group of exercises. The abdominal muscles are considered primarily antigravity or postural muscles. Hence, a little more endurance may be required. When doing abdominal work, most people do about 20 repetitions. Once you begin your strength-training program, you may use the form provided in Figure 3.16 at the end of this chapter to keep a record of your training sessions.

If time is a concern in completing a strength-training exercise program, ACSM recommends a minimum of one set of eight to twelve repetitions performed to near fatigue, using eight to ten exercises that involve the major muscle groups of the body (see Figure 3.17 at the end of this chapter). Training sessions should be conducted twice a week (see Figure 3.9). The recommendation is based on research showing that this training generates 70 to 80% of the improvements reported in other programs using three sets of about 10 RM.

FIGURE 3.9

Strength Training Guidelines*

Mode: 8 to 10 isotonic strength-training exercises involving the body's major muscle groups.

Resistance: Enough resistance to perform 8 to 12 repetitions to near fatigue

Sets: A minimum of one set

Frequency: At least twice a week

---

*Source: "The Recommended Quantity and Quality of Exercise for Developing and Maintaining Cardiorespiratory and Muscular Fitness in Healthy Adults by the American College of Sports Medicine," Med. Sci. Sports Exerc. 22:265-274, 1990.

MUSCULAR FLEXIBILITY

Improving and maintaining good joint range of motion throughout life is important in enhancing health and quality of life. Nevertheless, health care professionals and practitioners have generally underestimated and overlooked flexibility fitness.

The most significant detriments to flexibility are sedentary living and lack of physical activity. As physical activity decreases, muscles lose elasticity and tendons and ligaments tighten and shorten. Aging also reduces the extensibility of soft tissue, resulting in decreased flexibility.

Generally, flexibility exercises to improve joint range of motion are conducted following an aerobic workout. Stretching exercises seem to be most effective when a person is properly warmed up. Changes in muscle temperature can increase or decrease flexibility by as much as 20%. Cool temperatures have the opposite effect, decreasing joint range of motion. Because of the effects of temperature on muscular flexibility, many people prefer to do their stretching exercises after the aerobic phase of their workout.

Muscular Flexibility Prescription

The overload and specificity of training principles also apply to the development of muscular flexibility. To increase the total range of motion of a joint, the specific muscles surrounding that joint have to be progressively stretched beyond their accustomed length. Principles of mode, intensity, repetitions, and frequency of exercise also can be applied to flexibility programs.

Mode of Exercise

Three modes of stretching exercises promote flexibility: (a) ballistic stretching, (b) slow-sustained stretching, and (c) proprioceptive neuromuscular facilitation stretching.

Although all three types of stretching are effective in developing better flexibility, each has certain advantages.

Ballistic or dynamic stretching exercises require jerky, rapid, and bouncy movements that provide the necessary force to lengthen the muscles. This type of stretching helps to develop flexibility, but the ballistic actions may cause muscle soreness and injury because of small tears to the soft tissue.

Precautions must be taken to not overstretch ligaments, because they undergo plastic or permanent elongation. If the stretching force cannot be controlled, as in fast, jerky movements, ligaments can be easily overstretched. This, in turn, leads to excessively loose joints, increasing the risk for injuries, including joint dislocation and subluxation (partial dislocation). Most authorities, therefore, do not recommend ballistic exercises for flexibility development.

With the *slow-sustained stretching* technique, muscles are gradually lengthened through a joint's complete range of motion, and the final position is held for a few seconds. Doing a slow-sustained stretch causes the muscles to relax so that greater length can be achieved. This type of stretch causes little pain and has a low risk of injury. Slow-sustained stretching exercises are the most frequently used and recommended for flexibility development programs.

Proprioceptive neuromuscular facilitation (PNF) stretching has become more popular in the last few years. This technique, based on a "contract and relax" method, requires the assistance of another person (see Figure 3.10). The procedure is as follows:

1. The person assisting with the exercise provides initial force by slowly pushing in the direction of the desired stretch. The initial stretch does not cover the entire range of motion.

FIGURE 3.10

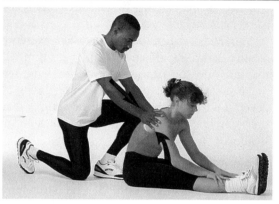

(a)

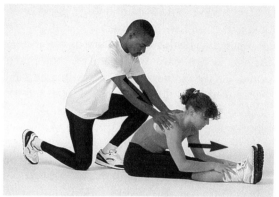

(b)

Proprioceptive neuromuscular facilitation stretching technique: (a) isometric phase, (b) stretching phase.

2. The person being stretched then applies force in the opposite direction of the stretch, against the assistant, who tries to hold the initial degree of stretch as closely as possible. An isometric contraction is being performed at that angle.

3. After 4 or 5 seconds of isometric contraction, the muscles being stretched are completely relaxed. The assistant then slowly increases the degree of stretch to a greater angle.

4. The isometric contraction is repeated for another 4 or 5 seconds; then the muscle(s) is relaxed again.

The assistant then can slowly increase the degree of stretch one more time. This procedure is repeated two to five times, until the exerciser feels mild discomfort. On the last trial, the final stretched position should be held several seconds.

Theoretically, with the PNF technique, the isometric contraction helps relax the muscle(s) being stretched, which results in greater muscle length. Although some fitness leaders believe PNF is more effective than slow-sustained stretching, the disadvantages are more pain with PNF, a second person is required to assist, and more time is needed to conduct each session.

Intensity of Exercise

Before starting any flexibility exercises, the muscles always should be warmed up using some calisthenic exercises. Higher body temperature can increase joint range of motion. Failing to do a proper warm-up increases the risk for muscle pulls and tears.

The intensity or degree of stretch when doing flexibility exercises should be only to a point of mild discomfort. Pain does not have to be a part of the stretching routine. Excessive pain is an indication that the load is too high and may lead to injury. Stretching should be done to slightly below the pain threshold. As participants reach this point, they should try to relax the muscle(s) being stretched as much as possible. After completing the stretch, the body part is brought back gradually to the starting point.

Repetitions

The time required in an exercise session for flexibility development is based on the number of repetitions performed and the length of time each repetition (final stretched position) is held. The general recommendation is that *each exercise should be done four or five times, holding the final position each time about 10 seconds.* As flexibility increases, the individual can gradually increase the time each repetition is held, to a maximum of one minute.

Frequency of Exercise

Flexibility exercises should be conducted five to six times a week in the initial stages of the program. After a minimum of 6 to 8 weeks of almost daily stretching, flexibility levels can be maintained with only two or three sessions per week, using about three repetitions of 10 to 15 seconds each. Figure 3.11 provides a summary of flexibility development guidelines.

Designing a Flexibility Program

To improve body flexibility, each major muscle group should be subjected to at least one stretching exercise. A complete set of exercises for developing muscular flexibility is presented in Appendix C. You may not be able to hold a final stretched position with some of these exercises (such as lateral head tilts and

---

FIGURE 3.11

Flexibility Development Guidelines

Mode:	Static stretching or proprioceptive neuromuscular facilitation (PNF)
Intensity:	Stretch to the point of mild discomfort
Repetitions:	Repeat each exercise 4 to 5 times and hold the final stretched position for 10 to 60 seconds
Frequency:	2 to 6 days per week

---

arm circles), but you should still perform the exercise through the joint's full range of motion. Depending on the number and the length of the repetitions, a complete workout will last between 15 and 30 minutes.

PREVENTION AND REHABILITATION OF LOW BACK PAIN

Few people make it through life without having low back pain at some point. An estimated 75 million Americans suffer from chronic low back pain each year. About 80% of the time, backache is preventable and is caused by: (a) physical inactivity, (b) poor postural habits and body mechanics, and (c) excessive body weight.

Lack of physical activity is the most common contributor to chronic low back pain. Deterioration or weakening of the abdominal and gluteal muscles, along with tightening of the lower back (erector spine) muscles, brings about an unnatural forward tilt of the pelvis (see Figure 3.12). This tilt puts extra pressure on the spinal vertebrae, causing pain in the lower back. Accumulation of fat around the midsection of the body contributes to the forward tilt of the pelvis, which further aggravates the condition.

Low back pain frequently is associated with faulty posture and improper body mechanics (body positions in all of life's daily activities, including sleeping, sitting, standing, walking, driving, working, and exercising). Incorrect posture and poor mechanics, as explained in Figure 3.13, increase strain not only on the lower back but on many other bones, joints, muscles, and ligaments as well.

The incidence and frequency of low back pain can be reduced greatly by including some specific stretching and strengthening exercises in the regular fitness program. In most cases, back pain is present only with movement and physical activity.

FIGURE 3.12

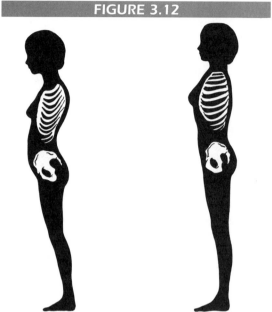

Incorrect (left) and correct (right) pelvic alignment.

If back pain is severe and persists even at rest, the first step is to consult a physician, who can rule out any disc damage and most likely will prescribe proper bed rest using several pillows under the knees for leg support (see Figure 3.13). This position helps release muscle spasms by stretching the muscles involved. In addition, a physician may prescribe a muscle relaxant or anti-inflammatory medication (or both) and some type of physical therapy. Once the individual is pain-free in the resting state, he or she needs to start correcting the muscular imbalance by stretching the tight muscles and strengthening the weak ones. Stretching exercises are always done first.

Several exercises for preventing backache and rehabilitating the back are given in Appendix D. These exercises can be done twice or more daily when a person has back pain. Under normal circumstances, three to four times a week is sufficient to prevent the syndrome.

GETTING STARTED AND STICKING TO AN EXERCISE PROGRAM

Starting and maintaining a fitness program is not easy if you are not accustomed to an exercise program. Introducing new behaviors into life's daily routine takes most people months to accomplish. A fitness program is no exception. Adding exercise to a person's lifestyle may require retraining (behavior modification).

Different things motivate different people to start and remain in a fitness program. Regardless of the initial reason for initiating an exercise program, you now need to plan for ways to make your workout fun. The psychology behind it is simple. If you enjoy an activity, you will continue to do it. If you don't, you will quit. Some of the following suggestions may help:

1. Start slowly. One of the most common mistakes people make with exercise is doing too much too quickly. This increases the risk for injuries and often leads to discouragement and exercise dropout. Keep in mind that the body's conditioning process takes months.

2. Select aerobic activities you enjoy doing. Picking an activity that you don't enjoy makes you less likely to keep exercising.

3. Combine various activities. You can train by doing two or three different activities the same week. This makes exercising less monotonous than repeating the same activity again and again.

4. Find a friend or group of friends to exercise with. Social interaction will make exercise more fulfilling. Besides, it's harder to skip if someone is waiting for you.

5. Set aside a regular time for exercise. If you don't plan ahead, it's a lot easier to skip. Holding your exercise hour "sacred" will help you adhere to the program.

FIGURE 3.13

Your Back and How to Care For It

HOW TO STAY ON YOUR FEET WITHOUT TIRING YOUR BACK

To prevent strain and pain in everyday activities, it is restful to change from one task to another before fatigue sets in. Housewives can lie down between chores, others should check body position frequently, drawing in the abdomen, flattening the back, bending the knees slightly.

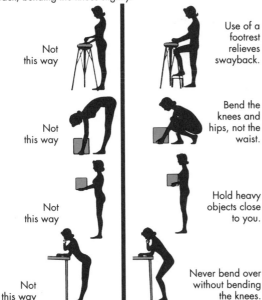

Not this way

Not this way

Not this way

Not this way

Use of a footrest relieves swayback.

Bend the knees and hips, not the waist.

Hold heavy objects close to you.

Never bend over without bending the knees.

HOW TO PUT YOUR BACK TO BED

For proper bed posture, a firm mattress is essential. Bedboards, sold commercially, or devised at home, may be used with soft mattresses. Bedboards, preferably, should be made of ¾ inch plywood. Faulty sleeping positions intensify swayback and result not only in backache but in numbness, tingling, and pain in arms and legs.

Incorrect:
Lying flat on back makes swayback worse

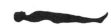

Use of high pillow strains neck, arms, shoulders

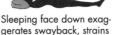

Sleeping face down exaggerates swayback, strains neck and shoulders

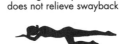

Bending one hip and knee does not relieve swayback

Correct:
Lying on side with knees bent effectively flattens the back. Flat pillow may be used to support neck, especially when shoulders are broad

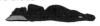

Sleeping on back is restful and correct when knees are properly supported

Raise the foot of the mattress eight inches to discourage sleeping on the abdomen

Proper arrangement of pillows for resting or reading in bed

HOW TO SIT CORRECTLY

A back's best friend is a straight, hard chair. If you can't get the chair you prefer, learn to sit properly on whatever chair you get. To correct sitting position from forward slump, throw head well back, then bend it forward to pull in the chin. This will straighten the back. Now tighten abdominal muscles to raise the chest. Check position frequently.

Relieve strain by sitting well forward, flatten back by tightening abdominal muscles, and cross knees.

Use of footrest relieves swayback. Aim is to have knees higher than hips.

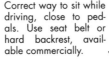

Correct way to sit while driving, close to pedals. Use seat belt or hard backrest, available commercially.

TV slump leads to "dowager's hump," strains neck and shoulders.

If chair is too high, swayback is increased.

Keep neck and back in as straight a line as possible with the spine. Bend forward from hips.

Driver's seat too far from pedals emphasizes curve in lower back.

Strained reading position. Forward thrusting strains muscles of neck and head.

6. Obtain the proper equipment for exercise. A poor pair of shoes, for instance, can increase the risk for injury, discouraging you right from the beginning.

7. Don't become a chronic exerciser. Learn to listen to your body. Overexercising can lead to chronic fatigue and injuries. Exercise should be enjoyable, and in the process you will need to "stop and smell the roses."

8. Exercise in different places and facilities to add variety to your workouts.

9. Conduct periodic assessments. Improving to a higher fitness category is a reward in itself.

10. Keep a regular record of your activities. This allows you to monitor your progress and compare it with previous months and years. Use forms similar to those in Figures 3.15 and 3.16 to monitor your aerobic and strength training programs.

11. See a physician if health problems arise. When in doubt, it's "better to be safe than sorry."

12. Set goals and share them with others. Quitting is tougher when someone knows what you are trying to accomplish. When you reach a specific goal, reward yourself with a new pair of shoes or a jogging suit.

SETTING FITNESS GOALS

Before you leave this chapter, you must consider your fitness goals. In the last few decades we have become accustomed to "quick fixes" with everything from super fast foods to one hour dry cleaning. Fitness, however, has no quick fix. Fitness takes time and dedication to develop, and only those who are committed and persistent will reap the rewards. Setting realistic fitness goals will help you design and guide your program. Figure 3.14 offers a goal-setting chart that will help you determine your fitness goals. Take the time, either by yourself or with your instructor's help, to fill it out.

As you prepare to write realistic fitness goals, base these goals on the results of your initial fitness test (pre-test). For instance, if your cardiovascular fitness category was poor on the pre-test, you should not expect to improve to the excellent category in a little more than 3 months.

Whenever possible, your fitness goals should be measurable. A goal that simply states "to improve cardiovascular endurance" is not as measurable as a goal that states "to improve to the good fitness category in cardiovascular endurance" or "to run the 1.5-mile course in less than 11 minutes." After determining each goal, you also will need to write measurable objectives to accomplish that goal. These objectives will be the actual plan of action to accomplish your goal. A sample of objectives to accomplish the previously stated goal for cardiovascular endurance development could be:

1. Use jogging as the mode of exercise.

2. Jog at 10:00 a.m. five times per week.

3. Jog around the track in the fieldhouse.

4. Jog for 30 minutes each exercise session.

5. Monitor heart rate regularly during exercise.

6. Take the 1.5-mile run test once a month.

Specific objectives will not always be met. Consequently, your goal may be out of reach. If so, reevaluate your objectives and make adjustments accordingly. If you set unrealistic goals at the beginning of your exercise program, be flexible with yourself and reconsider your plan of action but do not quit. Reconsidering your plan of action does not mean failure. Failure comes only to those who stop trying, and success comes to those who are committed and persistent.

FIGURE 3.14

Goal-Setting Chart

Indicate two or three general goals that you will work on during the next few weeks, and write the specific objectives you will use to accomplish each goal (you may not need eight specific objectives, write only as many as you need).

Cardiovascular Endurance Goal: _____

Specific Objectives:

1. _____

2. _____

3. _____

4. _____

5. _____

6. _____

7. _____

8. _____

Muscular Strength/Endurance Goal: _____

Specific Objectives:

1. _____

2. _____

3. _____

4. _____

5. _____

6. _____

7. _____

8. _____

(Continued)

FIGURE 3.14
Goal-Setting Chart (continued)

Muscular Flexibility Goal: _____

Specific Objectives:

1. _____

2. _____

3. _____

4. _____

5. _____

6. _____

7. _____

8. _____

Body Composition Goal: _____

Specific Objectives:

1. _____

2. _____

3. _____

4. _____

5. _____

6. _____

7. _____

8. _____

FIGURE 3.15

Aerobics Record Form

Date	Body Weight	Exercise Heart Rate	Type of Exercise	Distance In Miles	Time Hrs./Min.
1					
2					
3					
4					
5					
6					
7					
8					
9					
10					
11					
12					
13					
14					
15					
16					
17					
18					
19					
20					
21					
22					
23					
24					
25					
26					
27					
28					
29					
30					
31					
			Total		

FIGURE 3.15

Aerobics Record Form

Date	Body Weight	Exercise Heart Rate	Type of Exercise	Distance In Miles	Time Hrs./Min.
1					
2					
3					
4					
5					
6					
7					
8					
9					
10					
11					
12					
13					
14					
15					
16					
17					
18					
19					
20					
21					
22					
23					
24					
25					
26					
27					
28					
29					
30					
31					
			Total		

FIGURE 3.15

Aerobics Record Form

Date	Body Weight	Exercise Heart Rate	Type of Exercise	Distance In Miles	Time Hrs./Min.
1					
2					
3					
4					
5					
6					
7					
8					
9					
10					
11					
12					
13					
14					
15					
16					
17					
18					
19					
20					
21					
22					
23					
24					
25					
26					
27					
28					
29					
30					
31					
			Total		

FIGURE 3.15

Aerobics Record Form

Date	Body Weight	Exercise Heart Rate	Type of Exercise	Distance In Miles	Time Hrs./Min.
1					
2					
3					
4					
5					
6					
7					
8					
9					
10					
11					
12					
13					
14					
15					
16					
17					
18					
19					
20					
21					
22					
23					
24					
25					
26					
27					
28					
29					
30					
31					
			Total		

FIGURE 3.16

Strength Training Record Form

Name ____________________

Date

Exercise	St/Reps/Res*	St/Reps/Res*	St/Reps/Res*	St/Reps/Res*	St/Reps/Res*	St/Reps/Res*	St/Reps/Res*	St/Reps/Res*	St/Reps/Res*	St/Reps/Res*

* St/Reps/Res = Sets, Repetitions, and Resistance (e.g., 1/6/125 = 1 set of 6 repetitions with 125 pounds

FIGURE 3.16

Strength Training Record Form

Name ____________________

Date

Exercise	St/Reps/Res*	St/Reps/Res*	St/Reps/Res*	St/Reps/Res*	St/Reps/Res*	St/Reps/Res*	St/Reps/Res*	St/Reps/Res*	St/Reps/Res*	St/Reps/Res*

* St/Reps/Res = Sets, Repetitions, and Resistance (e.g., 1/6/125 = 1 set of 6 repetitions with 125 pounds

FIGURE 3.17

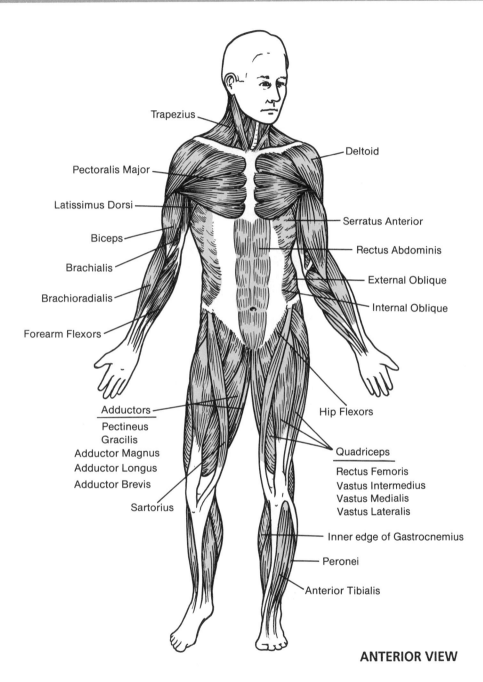

Trapezius

Deltoid

Pectoralis Major

Latissimus Dorsi

Serratus Anterior

Biceps

Rectus Abdominis

Brachialis

External Oblique

Brachioradialis

Internal Oblique

Forearm Flexors

Adductors
Pectineus
Gracilis
Adductor Magnus
Adductor Longus
Adductor Brevis

Hip Flexors

Quadriceps
Rectus Femoris
Vastus Intermedius
Vastus Medialis
Vastus Lateralis

Sartorius

Inner edge of Gastrocnemius

Peronei

Anterior Tibialis

ANTERIOR VIEW

Major Muscles of The Human Body (anterior view)

Fitness and Wellness

FIGURE 3.17

Fitness and Wellness

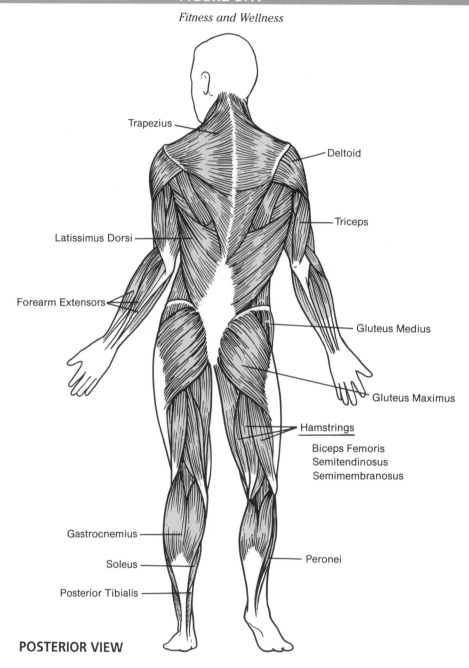

POSTERIOR VIEW

Major Muscles of The Human Body (posterior view)

Aerobic Activity Choices

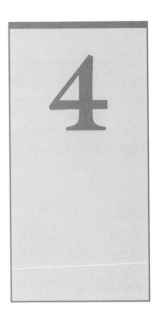

OBJECTIVES

- Learn the benefits and advantages of selected aerobic activities.
- Understand the sequence of a standard aerobic workout.
- Learn ways to enhance aerobic workouts.

One of the fun aspects of aerobic exercise is the many different choices of activities that promote cardiovascular development. You may select one or a combination of activities for your program. This choice should be based on personal enjoyment, convenience, and availability.

Most people pick and adhere to a single mode of exercise, such as walking, swimming, or jogging. No single activity develops total fitness. Many activities contribute to cardiovascular development. The extent of contribution to other fitness components is limited, though and varies among the activities. For total fitness, aerobic activities should be supplemented with strength (resistance) and flexibility exercise programs. Selecting a combination of aerobic activities (cross-training) nonetheless can add enjoyment to the program and keep exercise from becoming monotonous.

As you learn about the various activities in this chapter, keep in mind that your exercise sessions have to be convenient. So that you may enjoy exercise, select a time when you will not be rushed. A nearby location is recommended. People do not enjoy driving across town to get to the gym, health club, track, or pool. If parking is a problem, you may quickly get discouraged and use these factors as excuses not to stick to your exercise program.

WALKING

The most natural, easiest, safest, and least expensive form of aerobic exercise is walking (Figure 4.1). For years, many fitness practitioners believed that walking was not vigorous enough to improve cardiovascular functioning. Studies have established that brisk walking at speeds of 4 miles per hour or faster improves cardiovascular fitness.

From a health-fitness viewpoint, a regular walking program can significantly prolong life (see cardiovascular disease, Chapter 6). Although walking takes longer than jogging, the caloric cost of brisk walking is only about 10% lower than jogging the same distance.

Walking is perhaps the best activity to start a conditioning program for the cardiovascular system. Inactive people should start with one-mile walks four to five times per week. Walk times can be increased gradually by 5 minutes each week. Following 3 to 4 weeks of conditioning, people should be able to walk 2 miles at a 4-mile-per-hour pace, five times per week. For greater aerobic benefits, walk longer and swing the arms at a faster than normal pace. Light hand weights or a backpack (4 to 6 pounds) also add to the intensity of walking. Because of the additional load to the cardiovascular system, extra weights are not recommended for people who have cardiovascular disease.

Walking in water (chest-deep level) is an excellent form of activity for people with leg and back problems. Because of water buoyancy, individuals submerged in water to armpit level weigh only about 10 to 20% of their weight outside the water. The resistance the water creates as a person walks in the pool makes the intensity quite high, providing an excellent cardiovascular workout.

FIGURE 4.1

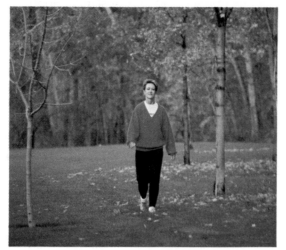

Walking: The most natural aerobic exercise.

HIKING

Hiking is an excellent activity for the entire family, especially during the summer and on summer vacations. Many people feel guilty if they are unable to continue their exercise routine during vacations. The intensity of hiking over uneven terrain is greater than walking (see Figure 4.2). An 8-hour hike can burn as many calories as a 20-mile walk or jog.

Another benefit of hiking is the relaxing effects of beautiful scenery. This is an ideal activity for highly stressed people who live near woods and hills. A rough day at the office can be forgotten quickly in the peacefulness and beauty of the outdoors.

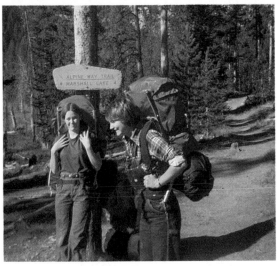

FIGURE 4.2

An 8-hour hike can burn as many calories as a 20-mile walk or jog.

JOGGING

Jogging is the most popular form of aerobic exercise. Next to walking, it is one of the most accessible and easiest forms of exercise. A person can find places to jog almost everywhere. The lone requirement to prevent injuries is a good pair of jogging shoes.

The popularity of jogging in the United States started shortly after publication of Dr. Kenneth Cooper's first Aerobics book in 1969. Jim Fixx's *Complete Book of Running* in the mid 1970s further contributed to the phenomenal growth of jogging as the predominant fitness activity in the United States.

Jogging three to five times a week is one of the greatest ways to improve cardiovascular fitness. The risk of injury, however, especially among beginners, is higher with jogging than walking. For proper conditioning, jogging programs should start with 1 to 2 weeks of walking. As fitness improves, walking and jogging can be combined, gradually increasing the jogging segment until it comprises the full 20 to 30 minutes.

Unfortunately, too many people abuse this activity. People run too fast and too long. Many joggers think that if a little is good, more is better. Not so with cardiovascular endurance. As indicated under "Frequency of Exercise" in Chapter 3, the aerobic benefits of training more than 30 minutes five times per week are minimal. Furthermore, the risk of injury increases greatly as speed (running instead of jogging) and mileage go up. Jogging approximately 15 miles per week is sufficient to reach an excellent level of cardiovascular fitness.

A good pair of shoes is a must for joggers. Many feet, knee, and leg problems originate from improperly fitting or worn-out shoes. A good pair of shoes should offer good lateral stability and not lean to either side when placed on a flat surface. The shoe also should bend at the ball of the foot, not at midfoot. Worn-out shoes should be replaced. After 500 miles of use, jogging shoes lose about a third of their shock absorption capabilities. If you suddenly have problems, check your shoes first. It may be time for a new pair. For safety reasons, joggers should stay away from high-speed roads, not wear headphones, and always run (or walk) against the traffic, so they will be able to see all oncoming traffic. At night, reflective clothing or fluorescent material should be worn on different parts of the body. Carrying a flashlight is even better because motorists can see the light from a greater distance than the reflective material.

An alternative form of jogging, especially for injured people, those with chronic back problems, or overweight individuals, is deep-water running (running in place while treading water). Deep-water running is almost as strenuous as jogging on land. In deep-water running, the land running motions are accentuated by pumping the arms and legs hard through a full range of motion. The participant usually wears a floatation vest to help maintain the body in an upright position. Many elite athletes train frequently in water to lessen the wear and tear on the body caused by long-distance running. These athletes have been able to maintain high oxygen uptake values through rigorous water running programs.

AEROBICS

Aerobics, formerly known as aerobic dance (see Figure 4.3) is thought to be the most common fitness activity for women in the United States. Aerobics involves a series of exercise routines performed to music. Routines include a combination of stepping, walking, jogging, skipping, kicking, and arm swinging movements. It is a fun way to exercise and promote cardiovascular development at the same time.

FIGURE 4.3

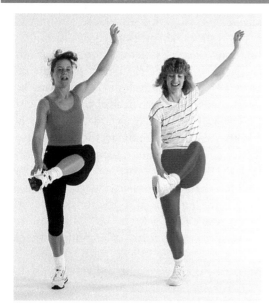

Aerobics: The most popular fitness activity for women in the United States.

The aerobics concept initially was developed in the early 1970s by Jacki Sorenson as a fitness program for Air Force wives in Puerto Rico. At first considered a fad, it now is a legitimate fitness activity with more than 20 million participants of all ages. Aerobics are now part of school curricula, health clubs, and recreational facilities.

High impact aerobics (HIA), the traditional form of aerobics, involves actions in which both feet may be momentarily off the floor at the same time. These movements exert a great amount of vertical force on the feet as they contact the floor. Proper leg conditioning through other forms of weight-bearing aerobic exercises (brisk walking and jogging), as well as strength training, are recommended prior to high-impact aerobic participation.

High impact aerobics is an intense activity, and it also produces the highest rate of aerobics injuries. Shin splints, stress fractures, low back pain, and tendinitis are all too common among high impact aerobics enthusiasts. These injuries are caused by the constant impact of the feet on firm surfaces. As a result, several alternative forms of aerobics have been developed.

In low impact aerobics (LIA) at least one foot is in contact with the floor or ground at all times, reducing the impact as each foot contacts the surface. The recommended exercise intensity is more difficult to maintain with low impact aerobics, though. To help elevate the exercise heart rate, all arm movements and weight-bearing actions that lower the center of gravity should be accentuated. Sustained movement throughout the program is also crucial to keep the heart rate in the target cardiovascular zone.

A relatively new form of aerobics is step aerobics (SA). Using a combination of stepping and arm movements, participants step up and down benches that range in height from 2 to 10 inches. Step aerobics adds another dimension to the aerobics movement and your exercise program. As previously noted, variety adds enjoyment to aerobic workouts. Step aerobics is viewed as a high intensity, but low impact activity. The intensity of the activity can be easily controlled by the height of the steps. Aerobic benches or plates are now commercially available. These plates can be safely stacked together to adjust the height of the steps. Beginners are encouraged to use the lowest stepping height available and then gradually advance to a higher bench. This practice will decrease the risk of injury. Even though one foot is always in contact with the floor or bench during step aerobics, this activity is not recommended for individuals with ankle, knee, or hip problems.

Other forms of aerobics include a combination of HIA and LIA, as well as moderate impact aerobics (MIA). The latter incorporates plyometric training. Plyometric aerobics requires forceful jumps or springing off the ground immediately after landing from a previous jump. This type of training is used frequently by jumpers (high, long, and triple jumpers) and athletes in sports that require quick jumping ability, such as in basketball and gymnastics.

With moderate impact aerobics, one foot is in contact with the ground most of the time. Participants, however, continually try to recover from all lower body flexion actions. This is done by quickly extending the hip, knee, and ankle joints without allowing the foot (or feet) to leave the ground. These quick movements make the exercise intensity of moderate impact aerobics quite high.

SWIMMING

Swimming is another excellent form of aerobic exercise. It uses almost all major muscle groups in the body, providing a good training stimulus for the heart and lungs.

Swimming is a great exercise option for individuals who cannot jog or walk for extended periods.

Compared to other activities, the risk of injuries from swimming is very low. The aquatic medium helps to support the body, taking pressure off bones and joints in the lower extremities and the back.

Maximal heart rates during swimming are approximately 13 beats per minute (bpm) lower than during running. The horizontal position of the body is thought to aid blood flow distribution throughout the body, thereby decreasing the demand on the cardiovascular system. Cool water temperatures and direct contact with the water seem to help dissipate body heat more efficiently, further decreasing the strain on the heart.

Fitness experts recommend that this difference in maximal heart rate (13 bpm) be subtracted prior to determining cardiovascular training intensities. For example, the estimated maximal swimming heart rate for a 20-year old would be 187 bpm ($220 - 20 - 13$).

To produce better training benefits, gliding periods such as those in the breast and side strokes should be minimized. Achieving proper training intensities with these strokes is difficult. The forward crawl is recommended for better aerobic results.

Overweight individuals need to swim fast enough to achieve an adequate training intensity. Excessive body fat makes the body more buoyant and often the tendency is to just float along. This may be good for reducing stress and relaxing, but it does not increase caloric expenditure to aid with weight loss. Walking or jogging in waist- or armpit-deep water are better choices for overweight individuals who cannot walk or jog on land for a long time.

With reference to the principle of specificity of training, swimming participants need to realize that cardiovascular improvements cannot be measured adequately with a walk/jog test. Most of the work with swimming is done by the upper body musculature. Although the heart's ability to pump a greater amount of oxygenated blood improves significantly with any type of aerobic activity, the primary increase in the ability of cells to utilize oxygen (VO_2 or oxygen uptake) with swimming occurs in the upper body and not the lower extremities. Therefore, fitness improvements with swimming are best attained by comparing changes in distances swum in a given time — say, 10 minutes.

WATER AEROBICS

Simple words best describe this relatively new form of exercise: fitness, fun, and safety for people of all ages (see Figure 4.4). Besides developing fitness, water aerobics provides an opportunity for socialization and fun in a comfortable and refreshing setting.

Water aerobics incorporates a combination of rhythmic arm and leg actions performed in a vertical position while submerged in waist- to armpit-deep water. The vigorous limb movements against the water's resistance during water aerobics provide the training stimuli for cardiorespiratory development.

The popularity of water aerobics as an exercise modality to develop the cardiovascular system has been on the rise in recent years. This increase in popularity can be attributed to several factors:

1. Water buoyancy reduces weight-bearing stress on joints and therefore reduces the risk for injuries.

2. Water aerobics is a more feasible type of exercise for overweight individuals and those with arthritic conditions who may not be able to participate in weight-bearing activities such as walking, jogging, and aerobics.

3. Heat dissipation in water is beneficial to obese participants who seem to undergo

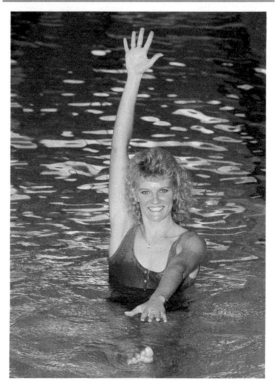

FIGURE 4.4

Water Aerobics: Fitness, fun, and safety for people of all ages.

a higher heat strain than average-weight individuals.

4. Water aerobics is available to swimmers and non-swimmers alike.

The exercises used during water aerobics are designed to elevate the heart rate, which contributes to cardiovascular development. In addition, the aquatic medium provides increased resistance for strength improvement with virtually no impact. Because of this resistance to movement, strength gains with water aerobics seem to be better than with most other land-based aerobic activities. Water exercises also help the joints move through their range of motion, promoting flexibility.

Another benefit is that weight reduction can be facilitated without pain and fear of injuries experienced by many who initiate exercise programs. Water aerobics provides a relatively safe environment for injury-free exercise participation. The cushioned environment of the water allows patients recovering from leg and back injuries, individuals with joint problems, injured athletes, pregnant women, and obese people to benefit from water aerobics. In water, these people can exercise to develop and maintain cardiovascular endurance and yet limit or eliminate the potential for further injury.

Similar to swimming, maximal heart rates achieved during water aerobics are lower than during running. The difference between water aerobics and running, however, is only 10 bpm (as compared to 13 for swimming). The smaller difference is thought to be related to the upright position maintained during water aerobics, which may not facilitate blood flow distribution to the same extent as during swimming. This difference of 10 bpm in maximal heart rate also should be considered when prescribing exercise intensities for water aerobics.

CYCLING

Cycling is an activity that most people learn in their youth. As a non-weight-bearing activity, it is a good exercise modality for people with lower body or lower back injuries. Cycling helps to develop the cardiovascular system, as well as muscular strength and endurance in the lower extremities. With the advent of stationary bicycles, this activity can be performed year-round.

Raising the heart rate to the proper training intensity is more difficult with cycling. As the amount of muscle mass involved during aerobic exercise decreases, so does the demand placed on the cardiovascular system. The thigh muscles do most of the work in cycling, making it harder to achieve and maintain a high cardiovascular training intensity.

Maintaining a continuous pedaling motion and eliminating coasting periods helps the participant achieve a higher heart rate. Exercising for longer periods also helps to compensate for the lower heart rate intensity during cycling. When comparing cycling to jogging, similar aerobic benefits take roughly three times the distance at twice the speed of jogging. Cycling, however, puts less stress on muscles and joints than jogging does, making the former a better exercise modality for people who cannot otherwise walk or jog.

To increase riding efficiency, the height of the bike seat should be adjusted so the legs are almost completely extended when the heels are placed on the pedals. The body, should not sway from side to side as the person rides. The cycling cadence also is important for maximal efficiency. Bike tension or gears should be set at a moderate level to be able to ride at 70 to 90 revolutions per minute.

Skill is important in road cycling (Figure 4.5). Cyclists must be in control of the bicycle at all times. They have to be able to maneuver the bike in traffic, maintain balance at slow speeds, switch gears, apply the brakes, watch for pedestrians and stoplights, and ride through congested areas. Stationary cycling does not require special skills. Nearly everyone can do it.

Safety is a key issue in road cycling. More than a million bicycle injuries occur each year. Proper equipment and common sense are necessary. A well-designed and maintained bike is easier to maneuver. Toe clips are recommended to keep feet from sliding and to maintain equal upward and downward force on the pedals.

Bike riders must follow the same rules as motorists. Many accidents happen because cyclists run traffic lights and stop signs. Some further suggestions are:

■ Use bike hand signals to let the traffic around you know of your actions.

FIGURE 4.5

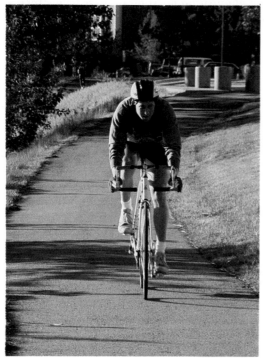

Skill is an important factor for safety and enjoyment of road cycling.

helmet for road cycling. Health and life are too precious to give up because of vainness and thriftiness.

■ Wear appropriate clothes and shoes. Special clothing for cycling is not required. Clothing should be lightweight and not restrict movement. Shorts should be long enough to keep the skin from rubbing against the seat. For greater comfort, cycling shorts have extra padding sewn into the seat and crotch areas. Experienced cyclists often wear special shoes with a cleat that snaps directly onto the pedal.

The stationary bike (see Figure 4.6) is the most popular piece of equipment sold by

FIGURE 4.6

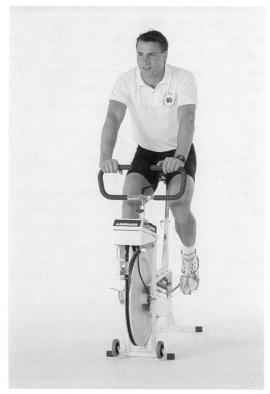

Exercising on a stationary bicycle adds variety to aerobic workouts.

■ Don't ride side by side with another rider.

■ Be aware of turning vehicles and cars backing out of alleys and parking lots; always yield to motorists in these situations.

■ Storm drains can cause unpleasant surprises if you do not cross them at the proper angle; front wheels can get caught and riders may be thrown from the bike.

■ Wear a good helmet, certified by the Snell Memorial Foundation or the American National Standards Institute. Many serious accidents and even deaths have been prevented by adequate helmet use. Do not allow fashion, aesthetics, comfort, or price to be a factor when selecting and using a

sporting good stores. Before buying a stationary bike, though, be sure to try the activity for a few days. If you enjoy it, you may want to purchase one. Invest with caution. If you opt to buy a lower-priced model, you may be disappointed. Good stationary bikes have comfortable seats, are stable, and provide a smooth and uniform pedaling motion. A sticky bike that is hard to pedal only leads to discouragement and, along with many others, ends up stored in the corner of a basement.

CROSS TRAINING

Cross training is training that combines two or more activities. This type of training is designed to enhance fitness, decrease injuries, and eliminate the monotony of single-activity programs. Cross training may combine aerobic and non-aerobic activities such as moderate jogging, speed training, and strength training.

Cross training can produce better workouts than a single activity. For example, jogging develops the lower body and swimming builds the upper body. Rowing contributes to upper body development and cycling builds the legs. Combining activities such as these provides good overall conditioning and at the same time helps to improve or maintain fitness. Cross training also offers an opportunity to develop skill and have fun with different activities.

Speed training is often coupled with cross training. Faster performance times in aerobic activities (running, cycling) are generated with speed or interval training. People who want to improve their running times often run shorter intervals at faster speeds than actual racing pace. For example, a person wanting to run a 6-minute mile may run four 440-yard intervals at a speed of 1 minute and 20 seconds per interval. A 440-yard walk/jog can become a recovery interval between fast runs.

Strength training is commonly used with cross training. Strength training helps to condition muscles, tendons, and ligaments. In many activities, improved strength enhances overall sports performance. For example, research has shown that although road cyclists who trained with weights showed no improvement in aerobic capacity, the cyclists had a 33% improvement in riding time to exhaustion when exercising at 75% of their maximal capacity.

ROPE SKIPPING

Rope skipping not only contributes to cardiovascular fitness, but it also helps to increase reaction time, coordination, agility, dynamic balance, and muscular strength in the lower extremities. At first, rope skipping may appear to be a highly strenuous form of aerobic exercise. Beginners often reach maximal heart rates after only 2 or 3 minutes of jumping. As skill improves, however, the energy demands decrease considerably.

Some people have claimed training benefits equal to a 30-minute jog in as little as 10 minutes of skipping. Although differences in strength and flexibility development are observed among different activities, 10 minutes at a certain heart rate provide similar cardiovascular benefits regardless of the nature of the activity. To obtain an adequate aerobic workout, the duration of exercise must be at least 20 minutes.

As with high impact aerobics, a major concern of rope skipping is the stress placed on the lower extremities. Skipping with one foot at a time decreases the impact somewhat, but it does not eliminate the risk for injuries. Fitness experts recommend that skipping be used sparingly and primarily as a supplement to an aerobic exercise program.

CROSS-COUNTRY SKIING

Many consider cross-country skiing as the ultimate aerobic exercise because it requires vigorous lower and upper body movements. The large amount of muscle mass involved in cross-country skiing makes the intensity of the activity very high, yet it places little strain on muscles and joints. One of the highest maximal oxygen uptakes ever measured (85 ml/kg/min.) was found in an elite cross-country skier.

In addition to being an excellent aerobic activity, cross-country skiing is soothing. Skiing through the beauty of the snow-covered countryside can be highly enjoyable. Although the need for snow is an obvious limitation, cross-country skiing simulating equipment for year-round training is available at many sporting goods stores.

Some skill is necessary for proficient cross-country skiing. Poorly skilled individuals are not able to elevate the heart rate enough to cause adequate aerobic development. Individuals contemplating this activity should seek out instruction to fully enjoy and reap the rewards of cross-country skiing.

IN-LINE SKATING

Frequently referred to as blading, in-line skating (see Figure 4.7) has become a highly popular fitness activity in recent years. Suddenly millions of children and adults are trying this activity. In the early 1990s, stores could not keep up with the demand for in-line skates.

In-line skating has its origin in ice skating. Because warm-weather ice skating was not feasible, blades were replaced by wheels for summertime participation. Four-wheel roller skates were invented in the mid 1700s, but the activity did not really catch on until the late 1800s. The first in-line skate with five wheels in a row attached to the bottom of a shoe was

FIGURE 4.7

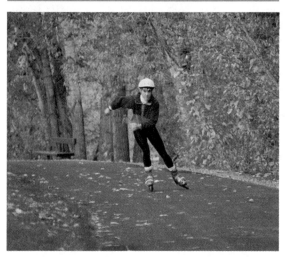

In-line Skating: A new fitness activity for the 1990s.

developed in 1823. The in-line concept took hold in the United States in 1980 when hockey skates were adapted for this road-skating.

In-line skating is an excellent activity to develop cardiovascular fitness and lower body strength. The intensity of the activity is regulated by how hard you blade. The key to effective cardiovascular training is to maintain a constant and rhythmic pattern, using arms and legs, and minimizing the gliding phase of blading. As a weight-bearing activity, in-line bladers also develop superior leg strength.

Instruction is necessary to achieve a minimum level of proficiency in this sport. Bladers commonly encounter hazards. Potholes, cracks, rocks, gravel, sticks, oil, street curbs, and driveways all pose challenges. Unskilled bladers are more prone to falls and injuries.

Good equipment will make the activity safer and more enjoyable. Blades range in price from $40 to $500. Recreational participants need not purchase the more costly competitive skates. An adequate blade should provide strong ankle support. Soft and flexible boots do not provide enough support. Small wheels offer more stability, and larger wheels enable greater speed. Blades should be purchased from stores that understand the sport and can provide sound advice according to skill level and needs.

Protective equipment is a must for in-line skating. Similar to road cycling, a good helmet that meets the safety standards set by the Snell Memorial Foundation or the American Standards Institute is important to protect yourself in case of a fall. Wrist guards and knee and elbow pads also are recommended. The kneecap and the elbows are easily injured in any fall. Nighttime bladers should wear light-colored clothing and reflective tape.

ROWING

Rowing is a low impact activity that provides a complete body workout. It mobilizes the use of most major muscle groups including the arms, legs, hips, abdominals, trunk, and shoulders. Rowing not only is a good form of aerobic exercise but, because of the nature of the activity (constant pushing and pulling against resistance), it also promotes total strength development.

To accommodate different fitness levels, workloads can be regulated on most rowing machines. Rowing, however, is not among the most popular forms of aerobic exercise. Similar to stationary bicycles, people should try the activity for a few weeks before purchasing a unit.

STAIR CLIMBING

If sustained for at least 20 minutes, stair climbing is an extremely efficient form of aerobic exercise. Precisely because of the high intensity of stair climbing, many people in our society stay away from stairs and instead ride elevators! Many people dislike living in two-story homes because they frequently have to climb the stairs.

Not too many places have enough flights of stairs to continuously climb for 20 minutes. Stair-climbing machines (Figure 4.8) offer an alternative. Stair climbing has become so popular that fitness enthusiasts often wait in line at health clubs to use the machines.

In terms of injuries, stair climbing seems to be a relatively safe exercise modality. Because the feet never leave the climbing surface, it is considered a low impact activity. Joints and ligaments are not really strained during climbing. The intensity of exercise is easily controlled because most stair climbers can be programmed to regulate the workload.

FIGURE 4.8

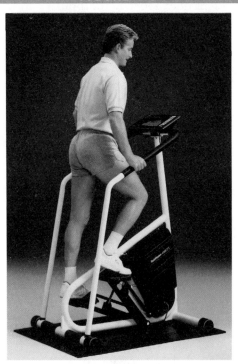

Stair climbing provides a rigorous aerobic workout.

(Photo courtesy of StairMaster® 4000 PT®.)

RACQUET SPORTS

In racquet sports such as tennis, racquetball (see Figure 4.9), squash, and badminton, the aerobic benefits are dictated by the individual's skill, intensity of the game, and how long the game is played. Skill is not only necessary to participate effectively in these sports but is also crucial to sustain continuous play. Frequent pauses during play do not allow people to maintain the heart rate in the appropriate target zone to stimulate cardiovascular development.

Many people who participate in racquet sports do so for enjoyment, social fulfillment, and relaxation. For cardiovascular fitness development, these people supplement the sport with other forms of aerobic exercise such as jogging, cycling, or swimming.

If a racquet sport is the primary form of aerobic exercise, participants need to try to run hard, fast, and as constantly as possible during play. They should not have to spend much time retrieving balls (bird or shuttlecock in badminton). Similar to low impact aerobics, all movements should be accentuated by

---

FIGURE 4.9

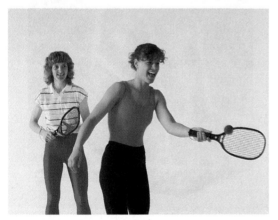

Racquet sports require rhythmic and continuous activity to provide aerobic benefits.

---

reaching out and bending more than usual, for better cardiovascular development.

RATING THE FITNESS BENEFITS OF AEROBIC ACTIVITIES

The fitness contributions of the aerobic activities discussed in this chapter vary among activities and individuals. As previously noted, the health-related components of physical fitness are cardiovascular endurance, muscular strength and endurance, muscular flexibility, and body composition. While an accurate assessment of the contributions to each fitness component are difficult to establish, a summary of likely benefits of these activities is provided in Table 4.1. Instead of a single rating or number, ranges are given for some of the categories. This is done because benefits derived are based on the person's effort while participating in the activity.

Regular participation in aerobic activities provides notable health benefits, including an increase in cardiovascular endurance, quality of life, and longevity. The extent of the cardiovascular development (improvement in VO_{2max}) depends on the intensity, duration, and frequency of the activity. The nature of the activity often dictates the potential aerobic development. For example, jogging is much more strenuous than walking. The effort during exercise also has an impact on the degree of physiological development. The training benefits of just going through the motions of a low impact aerobics routine, as compared to accentuating all motions (see low impact aerobics) are of a different magnitude.

Table 4.1 includes a starting fitness level for each aerobic activity. Attempting to participate in high intensity activities without proper conditioning often leads to injuries and discouragement. Beginners should start with low intensity activities that have a minimum risk of injuries. In some cases, such as in high impact

TABLE 4.1

Ratings for Aerobic Activities

Activity	Recommended Starting Fitness Level[1]	Injury Risk[2]	Potential Cardiovascular Endurance Development (VO_{2max})[3,5]	Upper Body Strength Development[3]	Lower Body Strength Development[3]	Upper Body Flexibility Development[3]	Lower Body Flexibility Development[3]	Weight Control[3]	MET Level[4,5,6]	Caloric Expenditure (cal/hour)[5,6]
Walking	B	L	1–2	1	2	1	1	3	4–6	300–450
Walking/Water/Chest-Deep	I	L	2–4	2	3	1	1	3	6–10	450–750
Hiking	B	L	2–4	1	3	1	1	3	6–10	450–750
Jogging	I	M	3–5	1	3	1	1	5	6–15	450–1125
Jogging/Deep Water	A	L	3–5	2	2	1	1	5	8–15	600–1125
High Impact Aerobics	A	H	3–4	2	4	3	2	4	6–12	450–900
Low Impact Aerobics	B	L	2–4	2	3	3	2	3	5–10	375–750
Step Aerobics	I	M	2–4	2	3–4	3	2	3–4	5–12	375–900
Moderate Impact Aerobics	I	M	2–4	2	3	3	2	3	6–12	450–900
Swimming (front crawl)	B	L	3–5	4	2	3	1	3	6-12	450–900
Water Aerobics	B	L	2–4	3	3	3	2	3	6-12	450–900
Stationary Cycling	B	L	2–4	1	4	1	1	3	6-10	450–750
Road Cycling	I	M	2–5	1	4	1	1	3	6-12	450–900
Cross Training	I	M	3–5	2–3	3–4	2–3	1–2	3–5	6–15	450–1125
Rope Skipping	I	H	3–5	2	4	1	2	3–5	8–15	600–1125
Cross-Country Skiing	B	M	4–5	4	4	2	2	4–5	10–16	750–1200
In-Line Skating	I	M	2–4	2	4	2	2	3	6–10	450–750
Rowing	B	L	3–5	4	2	3	1	4	8–14	600–1050
Stair Climbing	B	L	3–5	1	4	1	1	4–5	8–15	600–1125
Racquet Sports	I	M	2–4	3	3	3	2	3	6–10	450–750

[1] B = Beginner, I = Intermediate, A = Advanced

[2] L = Low, M = Moderate, H = High

[3] 1 = Low, 2 = Fair, 3 = Average, 4 = Good, 5 = excellent

[4] One MET represents the rate of energy expenditure at rest (3.5 ml/kg/min). Each additional MET is a multiple of the resting value. For example, 5 METs represents an energy expenditure equivalent to five times the resting value or about 17.5 ml/kg/min.

[5] Varies according to the person's effort (exercise intensity) during exercise.

[6] Varies according to body weight.

aerobics and rope skipping, the risk of injuries remains high despite adequate conditioning. Such activities should be used only to supplement training and are not recommended as the sole mode of exercise.

The MET range for the various activities is also included in Table 4.1. METS are an alternate method of prescribing exercise intensity and are frequently used by physicians who work with cardiac patients. One MET represents the body's energy requirement at rest or the equivalent of an oxygen uptake of 3.5 ml/kg/min. A 10-MET activity requires a ten-fold increase in the resting energy requirement or approximately 35 ml/kg/min. MET levels for a given activity vary according to the effort given by the individual. The harder a person exercises, the higher the MET level.

The effectiveness of the various aerobic activities in aiding with weight management is also provided in Table 4.1. As a general rule of thumb, the greater the muscle mass involved during exercise, the better the results. Rhythmic and continuous activities that involve large amounts of muscle mass are most effective in burning calories.

Higher intensity activities increase caloric expenditure as well. Increasing exercise time, however, compensates for lower intensities. If carried out long enough (45 to 60 minutes five to six times per week), even walking can be an excellent exercise mode for weight loss. Additional information on a comprehensive weight management program is given in Chapter 5.

TIPS TO ENHANCE YOUR AEROBIC WORKOUT

A typical aerobic workout is divided into three parts (see Figure 4.10):

1. A 2- to 5-minute warm-up phase during which the heart rate is gradually increased to the target zone.

2. The actual aerobic workout, during which the heart rate is maintained in the target zone for 20 to 60 minutes.

3. A 5- to 10-minute aerobic cool-down, when the heart rate is gradually lowered toward the resting level.

The exerciser should not stop abruptly following aerobic exercise. It will cause blood to pool in the exercised body parts, diminishing the return of blood to the heart. A lower blood return can cause dizziness or faintness, or even induce cardiac abnormalities.

To monitor the target training zone, you will need to check your exercise heart rate. As described in Chapter 2, check the pulse on the radial or the carotid artery. When taking the pulse at the carotid artery, be careful, because too much pressure on the artery may slow the heart and produce an inaccurate measurement.

When you check the heart rate, begin with zero and count the number of beats in a 10-second period, then multiply by 6 to get the per-minute pulse rate. You should take your exercise heart rate for 10 seconds rather than a full minute because the heart rate begins to slow down 15 seconds after you stop exercising.

Feeling the pulse while exercising is difficult. Participants should stop during exercise to check the pulse. If the heart rate is too low, increase the intensity of the exercise. If the rate is too high, slow down. You may want to practice taking your pulse several times during the day to become familiar with the monitoring techniques.

For the first few weeks of your program, heart rate should be monitored several times during the exercise session. As you become familiar with your body's response to exercise, you may have to monitor the heart rate only twice — once at 5 to 7 minutes into the exercise session and a second time near the end of

FIGURE 4.10

Typical Aerobic Workout Pattern

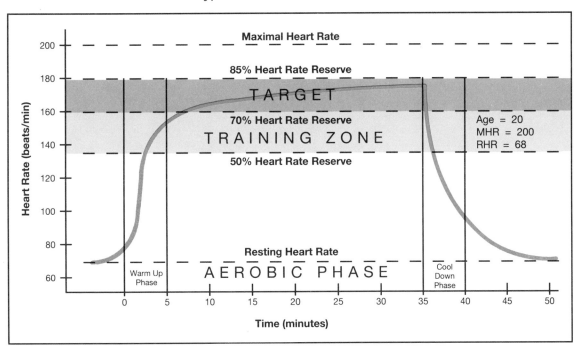

High cardiovascular endurance training zone

Moderate cardiovascular endurance training zone

the workout. To help you associate your perceived exertion of exercise and your heart rate, a form is provided in Figure 3.15 in Chapter 3.

Another technique sometimes used to determine your exercise intensity is simply to talk during exercise and then take the pulse immediately after that. Learning to associate the amount of difficulty when talking with the actual exercise heart rate will allow you to develop a sense of how hard you are working. Generally, if you can talk easily, you are not working hard enough. If you can talk but are slightly breathless, you should be in the target range. If you cannot talk at all, you are working too hard.

If you have difficulty keeping up with your exercise program, you may need to reconsider your objectives and start much more slowly. Behavior modification is a process. From a physiological and psychological point of view, you may not be able to carry out an exercise session for a full 20 to 30 minutes. For the first 2 to 3 weeks, therefore, you may just want to take a few 5-minute daily walks. As your body adapts physically and mentally, you then may gradually increase the length and intensity of the exercise sessions.

As a final point, learn to listen to your body. At times you will feel unusually fatigued or have much discomfort. Pain is the body's way of letting you know something is wrong.

If you have pain or undue discomfort during or after exercise, you need to slow down or discontinue your exercise program and notify the course instructor. The instructor may be able to pinpoint the reason for the discomfort or recommend that you consult your physician. You also are going to be able to prevent potential injuries by paying attention to pain signals and making adjustments accordingly.

Nutrition and Weight Control

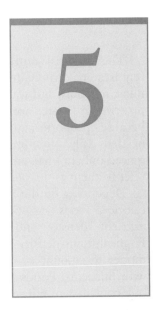

5

OBJECTIVES

- Define nutrition and describe its relationship to health and well-being.
- Learn the functions of nutrients in the human body.
- Become familiar with the various food groups and learn how to achieve a balanced diet.
- Learn to write and implement a sound weight control program.
- Identify myths and fallacies regarding nutrition and weight management.

The science of nutrition studies the relationship of foods to optimal health and performance. Although all the answers are not in yet, scientific evidence has long linked good nutrition to overall health and well-being. Proper nutrition means a person's diet is supplying all the essential nutrients to carry out normal tissue growth, repair, and maintenance. It also implies that the diet will provide enough substrates to produce the energy necessary for work, physical activity, and relaxation.

The typical American diet is too high in calories, sugar, fat, saturated fat, and sodium and not high enough in fiber. These factors all undermine good health. Overconsumption is a major concern for many Americans.

The essential nutrients the human body requires are carbohydrates, fats, protein, vitamins, minerals, and water. Carbohydrates, fats, protein, and water are termed *macronutrients* because proportionately large amounts are needed daily. Vitamins and minerals are required only in small amounts, and nutritionists refer to them as *micronutrients.*

Depending on the amount of nutrients and calories, foods can be classified into high-nutrient density and low-nutrient density. High-nutrient density foods contain a low or moderate amount of calories but are packed with nutrients. Foods that are high in calories but contain few nutrients are of low-nutrient density and are commonly called "junk food."

Carbohydrates are the major source of calories the body uses to provide energy for work, cell maintenance, and heat. They also help digest and regulate fat and metabolize protein. Each gram of carbohydrates provides the human body with 4 calories. The major sources of carbohydrates are breads, cereals, fruits, vegetables, and milk and other dairy products. Carbohydrates are divided into simple carbohydrates and complex carbohydrates. Simple carbohydrates (such as candy, soda, and cakes) are frequently denoted as sugars and have little nutritive value.

Complex carbohydrates are formed when simple carbohydrate molecules link together. Two examples of complex carbohydrates are starches and dextrins. Starches are commonly found in seeds, corn, nuts, grains, roots, potatoes, and legumes. Dextrins are formed from the breakdown of large starch molecules exposed to dry heat, such as when bread is baked or cold cereals are produced. Complex carbohydrates provide many valuable nutrients and can also be an excellent source of fiber or roughage.

Dietary fiber is a type of complex carbohydrate made up of plant material the human body cannot digest. It is present mainly in leaves, skins, roots, and seeds. Processing and refining foods removes almost all of the natural fiber. In our daily diets, the main sources of dietary fiber are whole-grain cereals and breads, fruits, and vegetables.

Fiber is important in the diet because it may help decrease the risk for cardiovascular disease and cancer. Several additional health disorders have been tied to low fiber intake, including constipation, diverticulitis, hemorrhoids, gallbladder disease, and obesity.

Fats, or lipids, are used in the body as a source of energy. They are the most concentrated energy source. Each gram of fat supplies 9 calories to the body. Fats also are part of the cell structure, used as stored energy and as an insulator to preserve body heat. They absorb shock, supply essential fatty acids, and carry the fat-soluble vitamins A, D, E, and K. The basic sources of fat are milk and other dairy products, and meats and alternates.

Proteins are the main substances the body uses to build and repair tissues such as muscles, blood, internal organs, skin, hair, nails, and bones. They are a part of hormones, enzymes, and antibodies and help maintain normal body fluid balance. Proteins also can be used as a source of energy but only if not enough carbohydrates and fats are available. The primary sources are meats and alternates and milk and other dairy products.

Vitamins are organic substances essential for normal bodily metabolism, growth, and development. Vitamins function as antioxidants, as coenzymes (primarily the B complex), which regulate the work of the enzymes; and vitamin D even functions as a hormone.

Based on their solubility, vitamins are classified into two types: fat-soluble vitamins (A, D, E, and K), and water-soluble vitamins (B complex and C). The body cannot manufacture vitamins. They can be obtained only through a well-balanced diet.

Vitamins C, E, beta-carotene (a precursor to vitamin A), and the mineral selenium serve as antioxidants, preventing oxygen from combining with other substances it may damage (see Figure 5.1). Oxygen is utilized during metabolism to change carbohydrates and fats into energy. During this process, oxygen is transformed into stable forms of water and carbon dioxide. A small amount of oxygen, however, ends up in an unstable form, referred to as *free radicals.*

Oxygen free radicals attack and damage proteins and lipids, in particular the cell membrane and DNA. This damage is thought to play a key role in the development of conditions such as heart disease, cancer, and emphysema (also see Chapter 6). Researchers believe that antioxidants offer protection by absorbing free radicals before they can cause damage and also by interrupting the sequence of reactions once damage has begun, thwarting certain chronic diseases.

Minerals are inorganic elements found in the body and in food. They serve several important functions. Minerals are constituents of all cells, especially those in hard parts of the body (bones, nails, teeth). They are crucial in maintaining water balance and the acid-base balance. They are essential components of respiratory pigments, enzymes, and enzyme systems, and they regulate muscular and nervous tissue excitability.

Water is the most important nutrient, involved in almost every vital body process. Water is used in digesting and absorbing food, in the circulatory process, in removing waste products, in building and rebuilding cells, and in transporting other nutrients. Water is contained in almost all foods but primarily in liquid foods, fruits, and vegetables. Besides the natural content in foods, every person should drink eight to ten glasses of fluids a day.

A BALANCED DIET

Most people would like to live life to its fullest, have good health, and lead a productive life. One of the fundamental ways to do this is through a well-balanced diet. As

---

FIGURE 5.1

Antioxidant nutrients, sources, and functions.

Nutrient	Good Sources	Antioxidant Effect
Vitamin C	Citrus fruit, kiwi fruit, cantaloupe, strawberries, broccoli, green or red peppers, cauliflower, cabbage	Appears to inactivate oxygen-free radicals
Vitamin E	Vegetable oils, yellow and green leafy vegetables, margarine, wheat germ, oatmeal, almonds, and whole grain breads, cereals	Protects lipids from oxidation
Beta-carotene	Carrots, squash, pumpkin, sweet potatoes, broccoli, green leafy vegetables	Soaks up oxygen-free radicals
Selenium	Seafood, meat, whole grains	Helps prevent damage to cell structures

illustrated in Figure 5.2, the recommended guidelines state that daily caloric intake should be distributed so about 58% of the total calories come from carbohydrates (48% complex carbohydrates and 10% sugar), less than 30% of the total calories from fat (equally divided [10% each] among saturated, monounsaturated, and polyunsaturated fats), and 12% of the total calories from protein (0.8 grams of protein per kilogram [2.2 pounds] of body weight). The diet also must include all the essential vitamins, minerals, and water.

One of the most detrimental health habits facing the American people today is the large amount of fat in the diet. Fat consumption in the average diet is about 37% of the total caloric intake; 30% or lower is recommended. To decrease the risk for disease, in particular cardiovascular disease and cancer, people must make a deliberate effort to decrease total fat intake. Therefore, being able to identify sources of fat in the diet is imperative to decrease fat intake.

As illustrated in Figure 5.3, each gram of carbohydrates and protein supplies the body with 4 calories, and fat provides 9 calories per gram consumed (alcohol yields 7 calories per gram). In this regard, just looking at the total amount of grams consumed for each type of food can be misleading.

For example, a person who consumes 160 grams of carbohydrates, 100 grams of fat, and 70 grams of protein has a total intake of 330 grams of food. This indicates that 33% of the total grams of food is in the form of fat (100 grams of fat ÷ 330 grams of total food × 100). In reality, almost half of the diet is fat calories.

In this sample diet, 640 calories are derived from carbohydrates (160 grams × 4 calories/gram), 280 calories from protein (70 grams × 4 calories/gram), and 900 calories from fat (100 grams × 9 calories/gram), for a total of 1,820 calories. If 900 calories are derived from fat, you can see that almost half of the total caloric intake is in the form of fat (900 ÷ 1,820 × 100 = 49.5%).

Realizing that each gram of fat equals 9 calories is a useful guideline when figuring out the fat content of individual foods. As shown in Figure 5.4, all you need to do is multiply

FIGURE 5.2

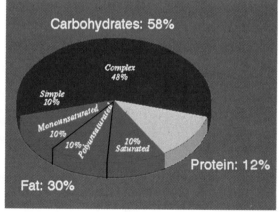

Current and recommended distribution of fat, carbohydrate, and protein intake expressed in percentages of total daily caloric consumption.

FIGURE 5.3

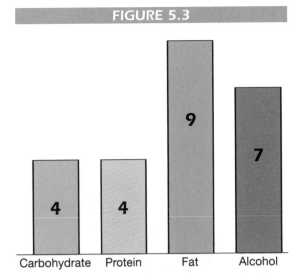

Calories per gram of food.

ANALYZING YOUR DIET

Achieving and maintaining a balanced diet is not as difficult as most people think. The Food Guide Pyramid contained in Figure 5.5, published by the U.S. Department of Agriculture, provides simple and sound instructions for nutrition. The pyramid contains five major food groups, along with fats, oils, and sweets, which are to be used sparingly. The daily recommended number of servings of the five major food groups are:

1. Six to eleven servings of the bread, cereal, rice, and pasta group.

2. Three to five servings of the vegetable group.

3. Two to four servings of the fruit group.

4. Two to three servings of the milk, yogurt, and cheese group.

5. Two to three servings of the meat, poultry, fish, dry beans, eggs, and nuts group.

As illustrated in the Food Guide Pyramid (Figure 5.5), grains, vegetables, and fruits provide the nutritional foundation for a healthy diet. Fruits and vegetables should include as a minimum one good source of

the grams of fat by 9 and divide by the total calories in that particular food. You multiply that number by 100 to get the percentage. For example, if a food label lists a total of 196 calories and 16 grams of fat, the fat content is 74% of total calories. This simple guideline can help you decrease fat in your diet.

FIGURE 5.4

Determining Fat Content in Food

Caloric Distribution for Creamy Peanut Butter

Serving size..........................	2 Tbsp
Calories	196
Protein................................	8 grams × 4 = 32 calories
Carbohydrates........................	5 grams × 4 = 20 calories
Fat....................................	16 grams × 9 = 144 calories
	Total calories = 196

Percent Fat Calories = (grams of fat × 9) ÷ calories/serving × 100

Percent Fat Calories in 2 Tbsp of Creamy Peanut Butter

$$[(16 \times 9) \div 196] \times 100 = 74\%$$

FIGURE 5.5

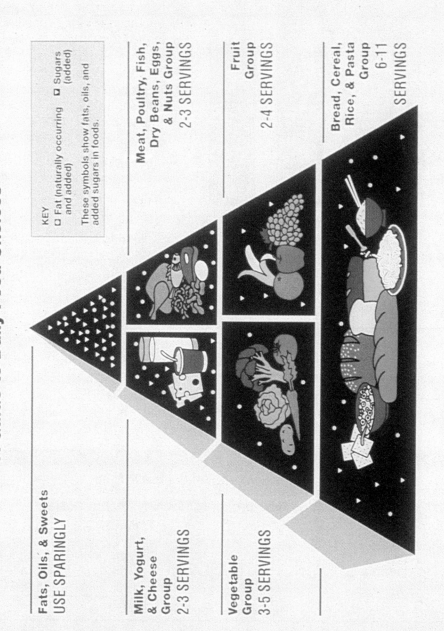

Food Guide Pyramid
A Guide to Daily Food Choices

KEY
□ Fat (naturally occurring   □ Sugars
and added)   (added)

These symbols show fats, oils, and
added sugars in foods.

Fats, Oils, & Sweets
USE SPARINGLY

Milk, Yogurt,
& Cheese
Group
2-3 SERVINGS

Meat, Poultry, Fish,
Dry Beans, Eggs,
& Nuts Group
2-3 SERVINGS

Vegetable
Group
3-5 SERVINGS

Fruit
Group
2-4 SERVINGS

Bread, Cereal,
Rice, & Pasta
Group
6-11
SERVINGS

What counts as one serving?

Breads, Cereals, Rice, and Pasta

1 slice of bread
1/2 cup of cooked rice or pasta
1/2 cup of cooked cereal
1 ounce of ready-to-eat cereal

Vegetables

1/2 cup of chopped raw or cooked vegetables
1 cup of leafy raw vegetables

Fruits

1 piece of fruit or melon wedge
3/4 cup of juice
1/2 cup of canned fruit
1/4 cup of dried fruit

Milk, Yogurt, and Cheese

1 cup of milk or yogurt
1-1/2 to 2 ounces of cheese

Meat, Poultry, Fish, Dry Beans, Eggs, and Nuts

2-1/2 to 3 ounces of cooked lean meat, poultry, or fish
Count 1/2 cup of cooked beans, or 1 egg, or 2 tablespoons of peanut butter as 1 ounce of lean meat (about 1/3 serving)

Fats, Oils, and Sweets

LIMIT CALORIES FROM THESE especially if you need to lose weight

> The amount you eat may be more than one serving. For example, a dinner portion of spaghetti would count as two or three servings of pasta.

A Closer Look at Fat and Added Sugars

The small tip of the Pyramid shows fats, oils, and sweets. These are foods such as salad dressings, cream, butter, margarine, sugars, soft drinks, candies, and sweet desserts. Alcoholic beverages are also part of this group. These foods provide calories but few vitamins and minerals. Most people should go easy on foods from this group.

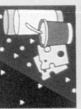

Some fat or sugar symbols are shown in the other food groups. That's to remind you that some foods in these groups can also be high in fat and added sugars, such as cheese or ice cream from the milk group, or french fries from the vegetable group.

When choosing foods for a healthful diet, consider the fat and added sugars in your choices from all the food groups, not just fats, oils, and sweets from the Pyramid tip.

How many servings do you need each day?

	Women & some older adults	Children, teen girls, active women, most men	Teen boys & active men
Calorie level*	about 1,600	about 2,200	about 2,800
Bread group	6	9	11
Vegetable group	3	4	5
Fruit group	2	3	4
Milk group	**2–3	**2–3	**2–3
Meat group	2, for a total of 5 ounces	2, for a total of 6 ounces	3, for a total of 7 ounces

* These are the calorie levels if you choose lowfat, lean foods from the 5 major food groups and use foods from the fats, oils, and sweets group sparingly.

** Women who are pregnant or breastfeeding, teenagers, and young adults to age 24 need 3 servings.

*Developed by the U.S. Department of Agriculture to promote a healthy diet for people in the United States.

vitamin A (apricots, cantaloupe, broccoli, carrots, pumpkin, dark leafy vegetables) and one good source of vitamin C (citrus fruit, kiwi fruit, cantaloupe, strawberries, broccoli, cabbage, cauliflower, green pepper).

Milk, poultry, fish, and meats are to be consumed in moderation. Skim milk and low-fat milk products are recommended. Three ounces daily of poultry, fish, or meat are advised, and no more than 6 ounces per day. All visible fat and skin should be trimmed off meats and poultry before cooking. A person should eat no more than three eggs per week.

The difficult part for most people is retraining themselves to adopt a lifetime healthy nutrition plan. If you (a) avoid excessive fats, oils, sweets, alcohol, and sodium, (b) increase your fiber intake, and (c) eat the minimum number of servings recommended for each of the five major groups in the Food Pyramid, you can achieve a well-balanced diet.

To aid you in balancing your diet, a form is given in Figure 5.6 for you to record your daily food intake. First, make as many copies as the number of days you wish to analyze. Whenever you eat something, record in Figure 5.6 the food and amount eaten. Recording this information immediately after each meal will enable you to more easily keep track of your actual food intake.

At the end of each day, consult the list of foods in Appendix B and record the code and number of calories for all foods consumed. Referring to Figure 5.6, record the number of servings under the respective food groups. If you eat twice the amount of a standard serving, double the calories and the number of servings.

You can evaluate your diet by checking whether you ate the minimum required servings for each food group. If you meet the minimum required servings at the end of each day, you are doing quite well in balancing your diet.

In addition to meeting the daily serving guidelines, a complete nutrient analysis is recommended to accurately rate your diet. A nutrient analysis can pinpoint potential problem areas in your diet, such as too much fat, saturated fat, cholesterol, sodium, and the like. A complete nutrient analysis can be quite an educational experience because most people do not realize how detrimental and non-nutritious many common foods are.

Analyzing your diet is quite simple if you utilize the computer software for this analysis.* To conduct the analysis, use the information you already have recorded on the form provided in Figure 5.6. Before running the software, fill out the information at the top of this form (age, weight, gender, activity rating, and number of days to be analyzed) and make sure the foods are recorded by the code and standard amounts given in the list of selected foods in Appendix B. Using the software, up to 7 days may be analyzed. The analysis covers calories, carbohydrates, fats, cholesterol, and sodium, as well as eight crucial nutrients: protein, calcium, iron, vitamin A, thiamin, riboflavin, niacin, and vitamin C. If the diet has enough of these eight nutrients, the foods (in natural form) consumed to provide these nutrients typically contain all the other nutrients the human body needs.

The computer-generated printout also includes the average daily nutrient intake and the recommended dietary allowance (RDA) comparison for all the above nutrients. A sample nutrient analysis printout is provided in Figure 5.7.

---

*Your instructor may have a copy of this software which is available through Morton Publishing Company in Englewood, Colorado.

FIGURE 5.6

Daily Diet Record Form

Date: _____

Name _____ Age: _____ Weight: _____ lbs.

Sex: _____ M _____ F   (Pregnant – P, Lactating – L, Neither – N)

Activity Rating: Sedentary (limited physical activity)   = 1
                Moderate physical activity   = 2
                Hard labor (strenuous physical activity) = 3

Number of days to be analyzed: _____   Day: _____ (1, 2 . . .)

No.	Code*	Food	Amount	Calories	Bread, Cereal, Rice & Pasta	Vegetable	Fruit	Milk, Yogurt & Cheese	Meat, Poultry, Fish, Dry Beans, Eggs, & Nuts
1									
2									
3									
4									
5									
6									
7									
8									
9									
10									
11									
12									
13									
14									
15									
16									
17									
18									
19									
20									
21									
22									
23									
24									
25									
26									
27									
28									
29									
30									
Totals									
Recommended Servings				**	6–11	3–5	2–4	2–3	2–3
Deficiencies									

Food Groups

**See list of nutritive value of selected foods in Appendix E.

**See Table 5.1

FIGURE 5.6

Daily Diet Record Form

Date: _____

Name _____ Age: _____ Weight: _____ lbs.

Sex: _____ M _____ F   (Pregnant – P, Lactating – L, Neither – N)

Activity Rating: Sedentary (limited physical activity)   = 1
                   Moderate physical activity   = 2
                   Hard labor (strenuous physical activity)   = 3

Number of days to be analyzed: _____   Day: _____ (1, 2 . . .)

No.	Code*	Food	Amount	Calories	Bread, Cereal, Rice & Pasta	Vegetable	Fruit	Milk, Yogurt & Cheese	Meat, Poultry, Fish, Dry Beans, Eggs, & Nuts
1									
2									
3									
4									
5									
6									
7									
8									
9									
10									
11									
12									
13									
14									
15									
16									
17									
18									
19									
20									
21									
22									
23									
24									
25									
26									
27									
28									
29									
30									
Totals									
Recommended Servings				**	6–11	3–5	2–4	2–3	2–3
Deficiencies									

**See list of nutritive value of selected foods in Appendix E.
**See Table 5.1

FIGURE 5.7

Computerized Nutritional Analysis*

```
NUTRIENT ANALYSIS
FITNESS & WELLNESS SERIES
by Werner W.K. Hoeger & Sharon A. Hoeger
Morton Publishing Company  -- Englewood, Colorado
```

Jane R. Moore   Date: 02-12-1992
Age: 20
Body Weight: 141 lbs (64.0 kg)
Activity Rating: Moderate

Food Intake Day One

Food	Amount	Calo-ries	Pro-tein gm	Fat gm	Sat Fat gm	Cho-les-terol mg	Car-bohy-drate gm	Cal-cium mg	Iron mg	Sodium mg	Vit A I.U.	Thi-amin mg	Ribo-fla-vin mg	Nia-cin mg	Vit C mg
Cocoa/hot/with whole milk	1 cup	218	9.1	9	6.1	33	26	298	0.8	123	318	0.10	0.44	0.4	2
Egg/scrambled w/milk butter	1 egg(s)	95	6.0	7	3.0	282	1	54	0.9	176	510	0.04	0.18	0.0	0
Bread/white	2 slice(s)	136	4.4	2	0.4	0	26	42	1.2	254	0	0.12	0.10	1.2	0
Butter	2 tsp	72	0.0	8	0.8	24	0	2	0.0	92	320	0.00	0.00	0.0	0
Milk/whole	1 c	159	9.0	9	5.1	34	12	288	0.1	120	350	0.07	0.40	0.2	2
Bread/whole wheat	2 slice(s)	122	5.2	2	1.2	0	24	50	1.6	264	0	0.12	0.06	1.4	0
Tuna/canned/oil/drained	1.5 oz.	84	12.5	4	0.9	30	0	4	0.8	69	35	0.02	0.05	5.1	0
Mayonnaise	2 tsp.	72	0.0	8	1.4	6	0	2	0.0	56	26	0.00	0.00	0.0	0
Pickles/dill	1 large	15	0.9	0	0.0	0	3	35	1.4	1,928	140	0.00	0.03	0.0	8
Potato/French fried	20 strips	428	6.8	20	3.4	0	56	24	2.0	10	0	0.20	0.12	4.8	32
Tomato sauce (catsup)	1 tbsp.	16	0.3	0	0.0	0	4	3	0.1	156	105	0.01	0.01	0.2	2
Apple/raw	1 med	80	0.3	1	0.0	0	20	10	0.4	1	120	0.04	0.03	0.1	6
Soda pop/root beer	12 oz.	140	0.0	0	0.0	0	36	17	0.2	45	0	0.00	0.00	0.0	0
Coleslaw	1 c	173	1.6	17	1.0	5	6	53	0.5	144	190	0.06	0.06	0.4	35
Spaghetti/meat balls/sauce	1 c	332	18.6	12	3.0	75	39	124	3.7	1,009	1,590	0.25	0.30	4.0	22
Pie/apple	1 pc. (3.5 in.)	302	2.6	13	3.5	120	45	9	0.4	355	40	0.02	0.02	0.5	1
Totals Day One		2,444	77.3	111	29.8	609	298	1,015	14.1	4,802	3,744	1.0	1.8	18.3	110

*Computer software available through Morton Publishing Company

FIGURE 5.7

Computerized Nutritional Analysis (continued)

NUTRITIONAL ANALYSIS: DAILY ANALYSIS, AVERAGE, AND
RECOMMENDED DIETARY ALLOWANCE (RDA) COMPARISON

	Calories	Protein gm	Fat %	Sat Fat %	Cholesterol mg	Carbohydrate %	Calcium mg	Iron mg	Sodium mg	Vit A I.U.	Thiamin mg	Riboflavin mg	Niacin mg	Vit C mg
Day One	2,444	77.3	40	11	609	48	1,015	14.1	4,802	3,744	1.0	1.8	18.3	110
Day Two	2,234	105.1	44	12	536	37	639	20.6	5,719	1,902	1.1	1.7	21.6	60
Day Three	2,491	92.0	43	19	603	43	1,787	14.7	3,919	6,351	1.6	3.5	18.2	55
Three Day Average	2,390	91.5	42	14	583	43	1,147	16.5	4,813	3,999	1.3	2.3	19.4	75
RDA	1,904*	51.2	<30	<10	<300	50)	1,200	15.0	1,904	4,000	1.1	1.3	15.0	60

*Estimated caloric value based on gender, current body weight, and activity rating (does not include additional calories burned through a physical exercise program).

OBSERVATIONS

Daily caloric intake should be distributed in such a way that 50 to 60 percent of the total calories come from carbohydrates and less than 30 percent of the total calories from fat. Protein intake should be about .8 to 1.5 grams per kilogram of body weight or about 15 to 20 percent of the total calories. Pregnant women need to consume an additional 15 grams of daily protein, while lactating women should have an extra 20 grams of daily protein (these additional grams of protein are already included in the RDA values for pregnant and lactating women). Saturated fats should constitute less than 10 percent of the total daily caloric intake.

Please note that the daily listings of food intake express the amount of carbohydrates, fat, saturated fat, and protein in grams. However, on the daily analysis and the RDA, only the amount of protein is given in grams. The amount of carbohydrates, fat, and saturated fat are expressed in percent of total calories. The final percentages are based on the total grams and total calories for all days analyzed, not from the average of the daily percentages.

If your average intake for protein, fat, saturated fat, cholesterol, or sodium is high, refer to the daily listings and decrease the intake of foods that are high in those nutrients. If your diet is deficient in carbohydrates, calcium, iron, vitamin A, thiamin, riboflavin, niacin, or vitamin C, refer to the statements below and increase your intake of the indicated foods or consult the list of selected foods in your textbook.

Caloric intake may be too high.

Total fat intake is too high.

Saturated fat intake is too high, which increases your risk for coronary heart disease.

Dietary cholesterol intake is too high. An average consumption of dietary cholesterol above 300 mg/day increases the risk for coronary heart disease. Do you know your blood cholesterol level?

Carbohydrate intake is low. Good sources of carbohydrates are whole grain breads and cereals, pasta, rice, fruits, and vegetables such as potatoes and peas.

Calcium intake is low. Good sources of calcium are milk, yogurt, cheese, green leafy vegetables, dried beans, sardines, and salmon.

Sodium intake is high.

Vitamin A intake is low. Foods high in vitamin A include skim milk fortified with vit. A, cheese, butter, fortified margarine, eggs (yolk), liver, and dark green/yellow fruits and vegetables.

Vitamin and Mineral Supplementation

Even though experts agree that in most cases vitamin and mineral supplements are not needed, people consume them at a greater rate than ever before. Research clearly shows that even when a person consumes as few as 1,200 calories per day, no supplementation is needed as long as the diet contains the recommended servings from the basic food groups.

For most people, vitamin and mineral supplementation is unnecessary and sometimes unsafe. Iron deficiency (determined through blood testing) is an exception, for women who have heavy menstrual flow. Some pregnant and lactating women also require supplements. In these instances, supplements should be taken under a physician's supervision.

Other people who may benefit from supplementation are alcoholics and street-drug users who do not have a balanced diet, smokers, strict vegetarians, individuals on extremely low-calorie diets, elderly people who don't regularly receive balanced meals, and newborn infants (usually given a single dose of vitamin K to prevent abnormal bleeding).

For healthy people with a balanced diet, supplementation provides no additional health benefits. It will not help a person run faster, jump higher, relieve stress, improve sexual prowess, cure a common cold, or boost energy levels.

Another fallacy about nutrition is that many people who regularly eat fast foods high in fat content or too many sweets think they need vitamin and mineral supplementation to balance their diet. The problem here is not a lack of vitamins and minerals but, instead, a diet too high in calories, fat, and sodium. Supplementation will not offset these poor eating habits.

EATING DISORDERS

Anorexia nervosa and bulimia are physical and emotional conditions usually arising from individual, family, or social pressures, in some combination, to become thin. These medical disorders are increasing steadily in most industrialized nations where society encourages low-calorie diets and thinness. People with eating disorders have an intense fear of becoming fat, which persists even when they lose a lot of weight.

Anorexia Nervosa

Anorexia nervosa is a condition of self-imposed starvation to lose and then maintain very low body weight. Approximately nineteen of every twenty anorexics are young women. An estimated 1 percent of the female population in the United States is anorexic. Anorexic individuals seem to fear weight gain more than death from starvation. Furthermore, they have a distorted image of their body and think of themselves as being fat even when they are emaciated.

Anorexics often come from a mother-dominated home. They may have a genetic predisposition, with other possible drug addictions in the family. The syndrome may begin following a stressful life event and their uncertainty about being able to cope effectively. The female role in society is changing more rapidly, and women seem to be especially susceptible. Life experiences such as gaining weight, starting menstrual periods, beginning college, losing a boyfriend, having poor self-esteem, being socially rejected, beginning a professional career, or becoming a wife or mother may trigger the syndrome.

These individuals typically begin a diet and at first feel in control and happy about the weight loss even if they are not overweight. To speed up the weight loss, they frequently combine extreme dieting with exhaustive exercise and overuse of laxatives and diuretics. Anorexics commonly develop obsessive and compulsive behaviors and emphatically deny the condition. They are constantly preoccupied with food, meal planning, grocery shopping, and unusual eating habits. As they lose weight and their health begins to deteriorate, anorexics feel weak and tired and may realize they have a problem, but they will not stop the starvation and they refuse to consider the behavior as abnormal.

Once they have lost a lot of weight and malnutrition sets in, physical changes become more visible. Some typical changes are amenorrhea (stopping menstruation), digestive problems, extreme sensitivity to cold, hair and skin problems, fluid and electrolyte abnormalities (which may lead to an irregular heartbeat and sudden stopping of the heart), injuries to nerves and tendons, abnormalities of immune function, anemia, growth of fine body hair, mental confusion, inability to concentrate, lethargy, depression, skin dryness, and lower skin and body temperature.

Many of the changes of anorexia nervosa can be reversed. Treatment almost always requires professional help, and the sooner it is started, the better the chances are for reversibility and cure. Therapy consists of a combination of medical and psychological techniques to restore proper nutrition, prevent medical complications, and modify the environment or events that triggered the syndrome. Seldom are anorexics able to overcome the problem by themselves.

Unfortunately, anorexics strongly deny their condition. They are able to hide it and deceive friends and relatives. Based on their behavior, many of them meet all of the characteristics of anorexia nervosa, but it goes undetected because both thinness and dieting are socially acceptable. Only a well-trained clinician is able to make a positive diagnosis.

Bulimia

Bulimia, a pattern of binge eating and purging, is more prevalent than anorexia nervosa. For many years it was thought to be a variant of anorexia nervosa, but now it is identified as a separate condition. It afflicts mainly young people, and as many as one in every five women on college campuses may be bulimic, according to some estimates. Bulimia also is more prevalent than anorexia nervosa in males.

Bulimics usually are healthy-looking people, well-educated, near recommended body weight, who enjoy food and often socialize around it. In actuality, they are emotionally insecure, rely on others, and lack self-confidence and esteem. Recommended weight and food are both important to them. As a result of stressful life events or the simple compulsion to eat, they periodically engage in binge eating that may last an hour or longer, during which they may consume several thousand calories. A feeling of deep guilt and shame follows, along with intense fear of gaining weight. Purging seems to be an easy answer, as the binging cycle can continue without the fear of gaining weight.

The most common form of purging is self-induced vomiting, and bulimics frequently ingest strong laxatives and emetics. Near-fasting diets and strenuous bouts of exercise are other typical practices. Medical problems associated with bulimia include cardiac arrhythmias, amenorrhea, kidney and bladder damage, ulcers, colitis, tearing of the esophagus and stomach, tooth erosion, gum damage, and general muscular weakness.

Unlike anorexics, bulimics realize their behavior is abnormal and feel great shame about it. Fearing social rejection, they pursue the binge-purge cycle in secrecy and during unusual hours of the day. Bulimia can be treated successfully when the person realizes this destructive behavior is not the solution to life's problems. A change in attitude can prevent permanent damage or death.

Treatment for anorexia nervosa and bulimia can be sought on most school campuses through the school's counseling center or the health center. Local hospitals also offer treatment for these conditions. Support groups, frequently led by professional personnel and usually free of charge, are available in many communities.

PRINCIPLES OF WEIGHT CONTROL

Achieving and maintaining ideal body weight is a major objective of a good physical fitness program. Unfortunately, only about 10% of all people who begin a traditional weight loss program (without exercise) are able to lose the desired weight. Worse, only one in 200 is able to keep the weight off for a significant time. Traditional diets have failed because few of them incorporate lifetime changes in food selection and exercise as the keys to successful weight loss.

Yet, fad diets continue to deceive people and promoters claim that the dieter will lose weight by following all the instructions.

Most diets are low in calories and deprive the body of certain nutrients, generating a metabolic imbalance that can even cause death. Under these conditions, a lot of the weight lost is in the form of water and protein, not fat.

Overly fat individuals who go on a crash diet lose nearly half the weight in lean (protein) tissue (see Figure 5.8). When the body uses protein instead of a combination of fats and carbohydrates as a source of energy, weight is lost as much as ten times faster. A gram of protein produces half the amount of energy that fat does. In the case of muscle protein, one-fifth of protein is mixed with four-fifths of water. Each pound of muscle yields only one-tenth the amount of energy of a pound of fat. As a result, most of the weight loss is in the form of water, which on the scale, of course, looks good.

Some diets allow only certain specialized foods. If people would realize that no "magic" foods provide all the necessary nutrients, and that a person has to eat a variety of foods to be well-nourished, the diet industry would not be as successful. Most of these diets create a nutritional deficiency, which at times can be fatal. The reason some of these diets succeed is that people eventually get tired of eating the same thing day in and day out and start eating less. If they achieve the lower weight without making permanent dietary changes, however, they quickly gain back the weight once they go back to old eating habits.

A few diets recommend exercise along with caloric restrictions — the best method for weight reduction, of course. A lot of the weight lost is because of the exercise, so the diet achieves its purpose. Unfortunately, if people do not permanently change their food selection and activity level, they quickly gain back the weight after discontinuing dieting and exercise.

Only a few years ago the principles governing a weight loss and maintenance program seemed to be fairly clear, but we now know the final answers are not in yet. Traditional concepts related to weight control have centered on three assumptions: (a) that balancing food intake against output allows a person to achieve recommended weight; (b) that fat people just eat too much; and (c) that the human body doesn't care how much (or little) fat is stored. Although these statements may contain some truth, they are still open to much debate and research.

Every person has a unique body fat percentage regulated by genetic and environmental factors. The genetic instinct to survive tells the body that fat storage is vital, and therefore it sets an acceptable fat level. This level

FIGURE 5.8

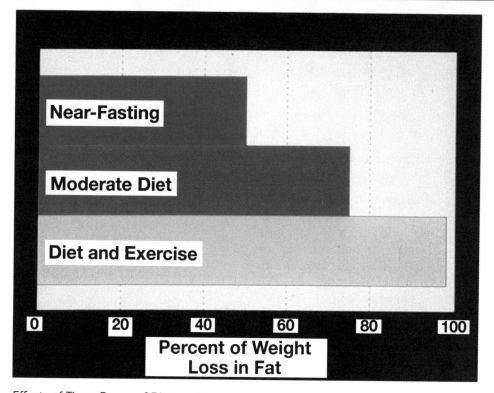

Effects of Three Forms of Diet on Fat Loss

Adapted from Shephard, R.J. *Alive Man: The Physiology of Physical Activity.* Springfield, IL: Charles C. Thomas, 484-488, 1975.

remains somewhat constant or may climb gradually because of poor lifestyle habits.

Under strict calorie reduction, the body may make extreme metabolic adjustments in an effort to maintain its fat storage. The basal metabolic rate may drop dramatically against a consistent negative caloric balance, and a person may be on a plateau for days or even weeks without losing much weight. When the dieter goes back to the normal or even below-normal caloric intake, at which the weight may have been stable for a long time, he or she quickly regains the fat loss as the body strives to regain a comfortable fat store.

Here's a practical illustration: Jim would like to lose some body fat and assumes that he has reached a stable body weight at an average daily caloric intake of 2,500 calories (no weight gain or loss at this daily intake). In an attempt to lose weight rapidly, he now goes on a strict low-calorie diet or, even worse, a near-fasting diet. Immediately the body activates its survival mechanism and readjusts its metabolism to a lower caloric balance.

After a few weeks of dieting at under 400 to 600 calories per day, the body now can maintain its normal functions at 1,500 calories per day. Having lost the desired weight, he terminates the diet but realizes the original intake of 2,500 calories per day will have to be lower to maintain the new lower weight.

To adjust to the new lower body weight, the intake is restricted to about 2,200 calories per day. Jim is surprised to find that even at this lower daily intake (300 fewer calories), weight comes back at a rate of about one pound every one to two weeks. After the diet ends, this new lowered metabolic rate may take several weeks or months to kick back up to its normal level.

From this explanation, individuals clearly should never go on very low-calorie diets. Not only will this decrease resting metabolic rate, but it also will deprive the body of basic daily nutrients required for normal function.

Under no circumstances should a person go on diets that call for below 1,200 and 1,500 calories for women and men, respectively. Weight (fat) is gained over months and years, not overnight. Equally, weight loss should be gradual, not abrupt. Daily caloric intakes of 1,200 to 1,500 calories provide the necessary nutrients if properly distributed over the various food groups (meeting the minimum daily required servings from each group). Of course, the individual has to learn which foods meet the requirements and yet are low in fat, sugar, and calories.

Furthermore, when a person tries to lose weight by dietary restrictions alone, lean body mass (muscle protein, along with vital organ protein) always decreases. The amount of lean body mass lost depends entirely on caloric limitation. When obese people go on a near-fasting diet, up to half of the weight loss can be lean body mass and the other half, actual fat loss. When the diet is combined with exercise, close to 100% of the weight loss is in the form of fat, and lean tissue actually may increase (see Figure 5.8). Loss of lean body mass is never good because it weakens the organs and muscles and slows down the metabolism.

Reductions in lean body mass are common in people who are on severely restricted diets. No diet with caloric intakes below 1,200 to 1,500 calories will prevent loss of lean body mass. Even at this intake level, some loss is inevitable unless the diet is combined with exercise. Many diets claim they do not alter the lean component, but the simple truth is that, regardless of what nutrients may be added to the diet, severe caloric restrictions always prompt a loss of lean tissue.

Too many people go on low-calorie diets constantly. Every time they do, the metabolic rate slows down as more lean tissue is lost. Many people in their 40s or older who weigh the same as they did when they were 20 think they are at recommended body weight. During this span of 20 years or more, they may have dieted too many times without participating in an exercise program. They regain the weight shortly after terminating each diet, but most of that gain is in fat. Maybe at age 20 they weighed 150 pounds of which only 15% to 16% was fat. Now at age 40, even though they still weigh 150 pounds, they might be 30% fat. They may feel that they are at recommended body weight, but wonder why they are eating so little and still having trouble staying at that weight.

Further, a diet high in fats and refined carbohydrates, near-fasting diets, and perhaps even artificial sweeteners will not allow a person to lose weight. On the contrary, these practices only contribute to fat gain. The only practical and sensible way to lose fat weight is through a combination of exercise and a diet high in complex carbohydrates and low in fat and sugar.

After studying the effects of proper food management, many nutritionists now believe the source of calories rather than the total number of calories should be the primary concern in a weight-control program. Most of the effort in this regard is spent in retraining eating habits, increasing the intake of complex carbohydrates and high-fiber foods, and decreasing the consumption of refined carbohydrates (sugars) and fats. In most cases, this change in eating habits brings about a decrease in total daily caloric intake.

A "diet" is no longer viewed as a temporary tool to aid in weight loss but, instead, as a permanent change in eating behaviors to ensure weight management and better health. The role of increased physical activity also must be considered because successful weight loss, maintenance, and recommended body composition are seldom attainable without a moderate reduction in caloric intake combined with a regular exercise program.

EXERCISE: THE KEY TO SUCCESSFUL WEIGHT MANAGEMENT

Perhaps the most significant factor in achieving ideal body composition is a lifetime exercise program. If a person is trying to lose weight, a combination of aerobic and strength training exercises works best. Because of the continuity and duration of aerobic exercise, it burns many calories. On the other hand, strength training has the greatest impact on increasing lean body mass.

The role of aerobic exercise in successful lifetime weight management cannot be underestimated. As illustrated in Figure 5.9, greater weight loss is achieved combining a diet with

FIGURE 5.9

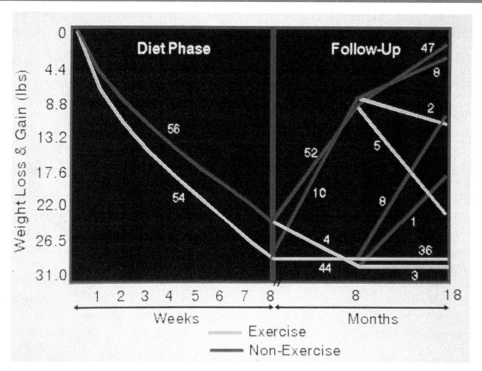

Value of aerobic exercise on weight loss and maintenance in moderately obese individuals (numbers in parenthesis indicate number of participants).

Source: Pavlou, K. N., S. Krey, and W. P. Steffe. "Exercise as an Adjunct to Weight Loss and Maintenance in Moderately Obese Subjects." *American Journal of Clinical Nutrition,* 49:1115-1123, 1989.

an aerobic exercise program. Of even greater significance, only the individuals who participated in an 18-month post-diet aerobic exercise program were able to keep the weight off. Those who discontinued exercise gained weight. Furthermore, all those who initiated or resumed exercise during the 18-month follow-up were able to lose weight again. Individuals who only dieted and never exercised regained 60% and 92% of their weight loss at the 6- and 18-month follow-up, respectively.

Faster weight loss can be obtained by combining aerobic exercise with a strength training program. Two exercise groups, a 30-minute aerobic group and a 15-minute aerobic plus 15-minute strength training (30 minutes total)

group participated in an 8-week, three-days-per-week study. Both groups followed a dietary plan that consisted of approximately 60% carbohydrates, 20% fats, and 20% proteins.

Results of the investigation showed that the aerobic group lost an average of 3½ pounds, 3 of which were fat, and the remaining 1/2 pound was lean tissue. The combined aerobic and strength training group lost an average of 8 pounds. Changes in body composition, however, indicated that the latter group actually lost 10 pounds of fat and gained 2 pounds of lean tissue (see Figure 5.10). These findings seem to indicate that a sensible strength training program is better to

FIGURE 5.10

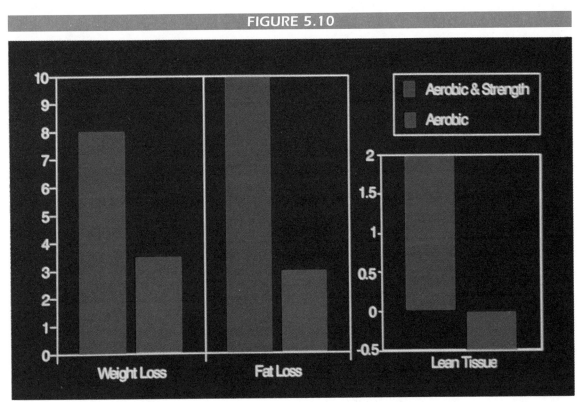

Changes in body composition through an aerobic exercise program and a combined aerobic/strength-training exercise program.

Source: Wescott, W. L. "You Can Sell Exercise for Weight Loss". *Fitness Management,* 7(12):33-34, 1991.

lose weight and maintain muscle mass and metabolic rate.

Another point of interest is that each additional pound of muscle tissue can raise the basal metabolic rate between 30 and 50 calories per day. Taking the conservative estimate of 30 calories per day, an individual who adds 5 pounds of muscle tissue as a result of strength training increases the basal metabolic rate by 150 calories per day, which equals 54,750 calories per year, or the equivalent of 15.6 pounds of fat. (One pound of fat represents approximately 3,500 calories.)

Because exercise promotes an increase in lean body mass, body weight often remains the same or even increases after beginning an exercise program, while inches and percent body fat decrease. More lean tissue means more functional capacity of the human body. With exercise, most of the weight loss becomes apparent after a few weeks of training, when the lean component has stabilized.

Research has revealed the fallacy of spot reducing or losing cellulite, as some people call the fat deposits that "bulge out" on certain body parts. These deposits are nothing but enlarged fat cells from accumulated body fat. Merely doing several sets of sit-ups daily will not get rid of fat in the midsection of the body. When fat comes off, it does so throughout the entire body, not just the exercised area. The greatest proportion of fat may come off the biggest fat deposits, but the caloric output of a few sets of sit-ups has almost no effect on reducing total body fat. A person has to exercise much longer to really see results.

Dieting never has been fun and never will be. People who are overweight and are serious about losing weight will have to make exercise a regular part of their daily life, along with proper food management and a sensible cut in caloric intake. Some precautions are in order, as excessive body fat is a risk factor for cardiovascular disease. Depending on the extent of

the weight problem, a medical examination and possibly a stress ECG (see Figure 2.2, Chapter 2) may be necessary before undertaking the exercise program. A physician should be consulted in this regard. Significantly overweight individuals also may have to choose activities in which they will not have to support their own body weight but will still be effective in burning calories. Joint and muscle injuries are common in overweight individuals who participate in weight-bearing exercises such as walking, jogging, and aerobics.

Better alternatives for overweight people are riding a bicycle (either road or stationary), water aerobics, walking in a shallow pool, or running in place in deep water (treading water). The last three modes of exercise are quickly gaining in popularity because little skill is required for participation. These activities seem to be just as effective as other forms of aerobic activity in helping individuals lose weight without the "pain" and fear of injuries.

One final benefit of exercise for weight control is that it allows fat to be burned more efficiently. Both carbohydrates and fats are sources of energy. When the glucose levels begin to drop during prolonged exercise, more fat is used as energy substrate. Equally important is that fat-burning enzymes increase with aerobic training. Fat is lost at a much faster rate by burning it in muscle. Therefore, as the concentration of the enzymes increases, so does the ability to burn fat.

DESIGNING YOUR OWN WEIGHT LOSS PROGRAM

In addition to exercise and adequate food management, sensible adjustments in caloric intake are recommended. Most research finds that a negative caloric balance is required to lose weight. Perhaps the only exception is in people who are eating too few calories. A nutrient analysis often reveals that "faithful" dieters are not consuming enough calories. These people actually need to increase their daily caloric intake (combined with an exercise program) to get the metabolism to kick back up to a normal level.

Referring to Figure 5.11 and Tables 5.1 and 5.2, you can estimate your daily caloric requirement. As this is only an estimated value, individual adjustments related to many of the factors discussed in this chapter may be necessary to establish a more precise value. Nevertheless, the estimated value does offer a beginning guideline for weight control or reduction.

The average daily caloric requirement without exercise is based on typical lifestyle

---

FIGURE 5.11

Computation Form for Daily Caloric Requirement

A. Current body weight   _____

B. Caloric requirement per pound of body weight (use Table 5.1)   _____

C. Typical daily caloric requirement without exercise to maintain body weight (A × B)   _____

D. Selected physical activity (e.g., jogging)*   _____

E. Number of exercise sessions per week   _____

F. Duration of exercise session (in minutes)   _____

G. Total weekly exercise time in minutes (E × F)   _____

H. Average daily exercise time in minutes (G ÷ 7)   _____

I. Caloric expenditure per pound per minute (cal/lb/min) of physical activity (use Table 5.2)   _____

J. Total calories burned per minute of physical activity (A × I)   _____

K. Average daily calories burned as a result of the exercise program (H × J)   _____

L. Total daily caloric requirement with exercise to maintain body weight (C + K)   _____

M. Number of calories to subtract from daily requirement to achieve a negative caloric balance**   _____

N. Target caloric intake to lose weight (L – M)   _____

---

* If more than one physical activity is selected, you will need to estimate the average daily calories burned as a result of each additional activity (steps D through K) and add all of these figures to L above.

** Subtract 500 calories if the total daily requirement with exercise (L) is below 3,000 calories. As many as 1,000 calories may be subtracted for daily requirements above 3,000 calories.

TABLE 5.1

Average caloric requirement per pound of body weight
based on lifestyle patterns and gender.

	Calories per pound	
Activity Rating	**Men**	**Women[1]**
Sedentary — Limited physical activity	13.0	12.0
Moderate physical activity	15.0	13.5
Hard Labor — Strenuous physical effort	17.0	15.0

[1] Pregnant or lactating women: Add three calories to these values.

TABLE 5.2

Caloric expenditure of selected physical activities
(calories per pound of body weight per minute of activity).

Activity*	Cal/lb/min	Activity	Cal/lb/min	Activity	Cal/lb/min
Aerobic Dance		Gymnastics		Stationary Cycling	
Moderate	0.075	Light	0.030	Moderate	0.055
Vigorous	0.095	Heavy	0.056	Vigorous	0.070
Archery	0.030	Handball	0.064	Strength Training	0.050
Badminton		Hiking	0.040	Swimming (crawl)	
Recreation	0.038	Jogging		20 yds/min	0.031
Competition	0.065	11.0 min/mile	0.070	25 yds/min	0.040
Baseball	0.031	8.5 min/mile	0.090	45 yds/min	0.057
Basketball		7.0 min/mile	0.102	50 yds/min	0.070
Moderate	0.046	6.0 min/mile	0.114	Table Tennis	0.030
Competition	0.063	Deep water**	0.100	Tennis	
Bowling	0.030	Judo/Karate	0.086	Moderate	0.045
Calisthenics	0.033	Racquetball	0.065	Competition	0.064
Cycling (level)		Rope Jumping	0.060	Volleyball	0.030
5.5 mph	0.033	Rowing (vigorous)	0.090	Walking	
10.0 mph	0.050	Skating (moderate)	0.038	4.5 mph	0.045
13.0 mph	0.071	Skiing		Shallow pool	0.090
Dance		Downhill	0.060	Water Aerobics	
Moderate	0.030	Level (5 mph)	0.078	Moderate	0.050
Vigorous	0.055	Soccer	0.059	Vigorous	0.070
Golf	0.030	StairMaster		Wrestling	0.085
		Moderate	0.070		
		Vigorous	0.090		

*Values are only for actual time engaged in the activity.   **Treading water
Adapted from:
  Allsen, P. E., J. M. Harrison, and B. Vance. *Fitness for Life: An Individualized Approach.* Dubuque, IA: Wm. C. Brown, 1989.
  Bucher, C. A., and W. E. Prentice, *Fitness for College and Life.* St. Louis: Times Mirror/Mosby College Publishing, 1989.
  Consolazio, C. F., R. E. Johnson, and L. J. Pecora. *Physiological measurements of Metabolic Functions in Man.* New York: McGraw-Hill, 1963.
  Hockey, R. V. *Physical Fitness: The Pathway to Healthful Living.* St. Louis: Times Mirror/Mosby College Publishing, 1989.

patterns, total body weight, and gender. Individuals who hold jobs that require heavy manual labor burn more calories during the day than those who have sedentary jobs (such as working behind a desk). To find your activity level, refer to Table 5.1 and rate yourself accordingly. The number given in Table 5.1 is per pound of body weight, so you multiply your current weight by that number. For example, the typical caloric requirement to maintain body weight for a moderately active male who weighs 160 pounds is 2,400 calories (160 lbs × 15 cal/lb).

The second step is to determine the average number of calories burned on a daily basis as a result of exercise. To get this number, figure out the total number of minutes you exercise weekly, and then figure the daily average exercise time. For instance, a person cycling at thirteen miles per hour, five times a week, thirty minutes each time, exercises 150 minutes per week (5 × 30). The average daily exercise time would be 21 minutes (150 ÷ 7 and round off to the lowest unit).

Next, from Table 5.2, find the energy requirement for the activity (or activities) chosen for the exercise program. In the case of cycling (13 miles per hour), the requirement is .071 calories per pound of body weight per minute of activity (cal/lb/min). With a body weight of 160 pounds, this man would burn 11.4 calories each minute (body weight × .071, or 160 × .071). In 21 minutes, he burns approximately 240 calories (21 × 11.4).

The third step is to obtain the estimated total caloric requirement, with exercise, needed to maintain body weight. To do this, add the typical daily requirement (without exercise) and the average calories burned through exercise. In our example, it is 2,640 calories (2,400 + 240).

If a negative caloric balance is recommended to lose weight, this person has to consume fewer than 2,640 daily calories to achieve the objective. Because of the many factors that play a role in weight control, the previous value is only an estimated daily requirement. Furthermore, to lose weight, we cannot predict that you will lose exactly one pound of fat in one week if you cut daily intake by 500 calories (500 × 7 = 3,500 calories, or the equivalent of one pound of fat).

The estimated daily caloric figure is only a target guideline for weight control. Periodic readjustments are necessary because individuals differ, and the estimated daily cost changes as you lose weight and modify your exercise habits.

The recommended number of calories to subtract from the daily intake and thereby obtain a negative caloric balance depends on the typical daily requirement. At this point, the best recommendation is to moderately decrease the daily intake, never below 1,200 calories for women and 1,500 for men.

A good rule to follow is to restrict the intake by no more than 500 calories if the daily requirement is below 3,000 calories. For caloric requirements of more than 3,000, as many as 1,000 calories per day may be subtracted from the total intake. The daily distribution should be approximately 60% carbohydrates (mostly complex carbohydrates), less than 30% fat, and about 12% protein.

The time of day when food is consumed also may play a part in weight reduction. A study conducted at the Aerobics Research Center in Dallas, Texas, indicated that when a person is on a diet, weight is lost most effectively if he or she consumes most of the calories before 1:00 p.m. and not during the evening meal. This center recommends that when a person is attempting to lose weight, intake should consist of a minimum of 25% of the total daily calories for breakfast, 50% for lunch, and 25% or less at dinner.

Other experts have reported that if most of the daily calories are consumed during one meal, the body may perceive that something is wrong and will slow down the metabolism so it can store a greater amount of calories in the form of fat. Also, eating most of the calories in one meal causes a person to go hungry the rest of the day, making it harder to adhere to the diet.

TIPS TO HELP CHANGE BEHAVIOR AND ADHERE TO A LIFETIME WEIGHT MANAGEMENT PROGRAM

Achieving and maintaining recommended body composition is by no means impossible, but it does require desire and commitment. If adequate weight management is to become a reality, some retraining of behavior is crucial for success. Modifying old habits and developing new positive behaviors take time. Individuals have applied the following management techniques to successfully change detrimental behavior and adhere to a positive lifetime weight control program.

In developing a retraining program, people are not expected to use all of the strategies listed but should check the ones that apply to them.

1. **Have a commitment to change.** The first necessary ingredient to modify behavior is the desire to do so. The reasons for change must be more compelling than those for continuing present lifestyle patterns. People must accept that they have a problem and decide by themselves whether they really want to change. If they are sincerely committed, the chances for success are enhanced already.

2. **Set realistic goals.** Most people with a weight problem would like to lose weight in a relatively short time but fail to realize that the weight problem developed over a span of several years. A sound weight reduction and maintenance program can be accomplished only by establishing new lifetime eating and exercise habits, both of which take time to develop.

    In setting a realistic long-term goal, short-term objectives also should be planned. The long-term goal may be a decrease body fat to 20% of total body weight. The short-term objective may be a 1% decrease in body fat each month. Objectives like these allow for regular evaluation and help maintain motivation and renewed commitment to attain the long-term goal.

3. **Incorporate exercise into the program.** Choosing enjoyable activities, places, times, equipment, and people to work with helps a person adhere to an exercise program. Details on developing a complete exercise program are included in Chapter 3.

4. **Develop healthy eating patterns.** The individual should plan on eating three regular meals per day consistent with the body's nutritional requirements, and learn to differentiate hunger from appetite. Hunger is the actual physical need for food. Appetite is a desire for food, usually triggered by factors such as stress, habit, boredom, depression, food availability, or just the thought of food itself. Individuals should eat only when they have a physical need. In this regard, developing and sticking to a regular meal pattern helps control hunger.

5. **Avoid automatic eating.** Many people associate certain daily activities with eating. For example, people eat while cooking, watching television, reading, talking on the telephone, or visiting with

neighbors. Most of the time, the foods consumed in these situations lack nutritional value or are high in sugar and fat.

6. **Stay busy.** People tend to eat more when they sit around and do nothing. Occupying the mind and body with activities not associated with eating helps take away the desire to eat. Walking, cycling, playing sports, gardening, sewing, or visiting a library, a museum, a park are some options. People might develop other skills and interests or try something new and exciting to break the routine of life.

7. **Plan meals ahead of time.** Sensible shopping is essential to accomplish this objective (by the way, shop on a full stomach, because hungry shoppers tend to impulsively buy unhealthy foods — and then snack on the way home). The shopping list should include whole-grain breads and cereals, fruits and vegetables, low-fat milk and dairy products, lean meats, fish, and poultry.

8. **Cook wisely.** Specifically:

   — Use less fat and refined foods in food preparation.

   — Trim all visible fat off meats and remove skin from poultry before cooking.

   — Skim the fat off gravies and soups.

   — Bake, broil, and boil instead of frying.

   — Sparingly use butter, cream, mayonnaise, and salad dressings.

   — Avoid coconut oil, palm oil, and cocoa butter.

   — Prepare plenty of bulky foods.

   — Add whole-grain breads and cereals, vegetables, and legumes to most meals.

   — Try fruits for dessert.

   — Beware of soda pop, fruit juices, and fruit-flavored drinks.

   — In addition to sugar, cut down on other refined carbohydrates such as corn syrup, malt sugar, dextrose, and fructose.

   — Drink plenty of water — at least six glasses a day.

9. **Do not serve more food than you should eat.** The food should be measured in portions, and serving dishes should be kept away from the table. This means you will eat less, have a harder time getting seconds, and have less appetite because the food is not visible. People should not be forced to eat when they are satisfied (including children after they already have had a healthy, nutritious serving).

10. **Learn to eat slowly and at the table only.** Eating is one of the pleasures of life, and we need to take time to enjoy it. Eating on the run is not good because the body doesn't have enough time to "register" nutritive and caloric consumption and people overeat before the body perceives the fullness signal. Always eating at the table also forces people to take time out to eat, and it deters snacking between meals, primarily because of the extra time and effort required to sit down and eat. When people are done eating, they should not sit around the table but, rather, clean up and put away the food to keep from unnecessary snacking.

11. **Avoid social binges.** Social gatherings tend to entice self-defeating behavior. Visual imagery might help before attending any social gatherings: Plan ahead and visualize yourself in that gathering. Do

not feel pressured to eat or drink, and don't rationalize in these situations. Choose low-calorie foods, and entertain yourself with other activities such as dancing and talking.

12. **Refrain from raiding the refrigerator and the cookie jar.** In these tempting situations, people should take control, stop and think what is happening. Environmental management is another tactic: Do not bring high-calorie, high-sugar, or high-fat foods into the house. If they are already there, they should be stored where they are hard to get to or see. If they are out of sight or not readily available, the temptation is less. Keeping food in places such as the garage and basement tends to discourage people from taking the time and effort to get them. By no means should you have to completely eliminate treats, but all things should be done in moderation.

13. **Practice stress management techniques.** Many people snack and increase food consumption in stressful situations. Eating is not a stress-releasing activity and instead can aggravate the problem if weight control is an issue.

14. **Monitor changes and reward accomplishments.** Feedback on fat loss, lean tissue gain, and weight loss is a reward in itself. Awareness of changes in body composition also helps reinforce new behaviors. Being able to exercise without interruption for 15, 20, 30, 60 minutes, swimming a certain distance, running a

mile — all these accomplishments deserve recognition. Meeting objectives calls for rewards, but not related to eating — new clothing, a tennis racquet, a bicycle, exercise shoes, or something else that is special and you would not have acquired otherwise.

15. **Think positive.** Negative thoughts about how difficult changing past behaviors might be are detracting. It's better to think of the benefits you will reap, such as feeling, looking, and functioning better, plus enjoying better health and improving the quality of life. Negative environments and people who will not be supportive should be avoided.

IN CONCLUSION

There is no simple and quick way to take off excessive body fat and keep it off for good. Weight management is accomplished through a lifetime commitment to physical activity and proper food selection. When taking part in a weight (fat) reduction program, people also have to moderately decrease their caloric intake and implement strategies to modify unhealthy eating behaviors. During the process of behavior modification, relapses into past negative behaviors are almost inevitable. Making mistakes is human and does not necessarily mean failure. Failure comes to those who give up and do not use previous experiences to build upon and, instead, develop skills that will prevent self-defeating behaviors in the future. "Where there's a will, there's a way," and those who persist will reap the rewards.

A Healthy Lifestyle Approach

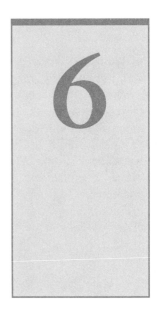

6

OBJECTIVES

- Learn the importance of implementing a healthy lifestyle program.
- Understand the major risk factors for coronary heart disease.
- Become acquainted with cancer prevention guidelines.
- Learn how to cope with stress.
- Recognize the relationship between spirituality and wellness.
- Learn the health consequences of chemical abuse and irresponsible sex.

Although people in the United States believe firmly in the benefits of physical activity and positive lifestyle habits as a means to promote better health, most do not reap these benefits because they simply do not know how to put into practice a sound fitness and wellness program that will yield the desired results. Unfortunately, many of the present lifestyle patterns of the American people are such a serious threat to our health that they actually increase the deterioration rate of the human body and lead to premature illness and mortality. Improving the quality and most likely the longevity of our lives is a matter of personal choice. Experts term the combination of a fitness program and a healthy lifestyle program the "wellness approach" to better health and quality of life.

Wellness is defined as the constant and deliberate effort to stay healthy and achieve the highest potential for well-being. Wellness incorporates healthy lifestyle factors such as adequate fitness, proper nutrition, stress management, disease prevention, spirituality, smoking cessation, personal safety, substance abuse control, regular physical examinations, health education, and environmental support (Figure 6.1).

The difference between physical fitness and wellness is best illustrated in the following example. An individual who runs 3 miles a day, lifts weights regularly, participates in stretching exercises, and watches his or her body weight can easily be classified in the good or excellent category for each of the fitness components. If this same individual, however, has high blood pressure, smokes, is under constant stress, consumes too much alcohol, and eats too many fatty foods, he or she is probably developing several risk factors for cardiovascular disease and may not be aware of it. A *risk factor* is an

FIGURE 6.1

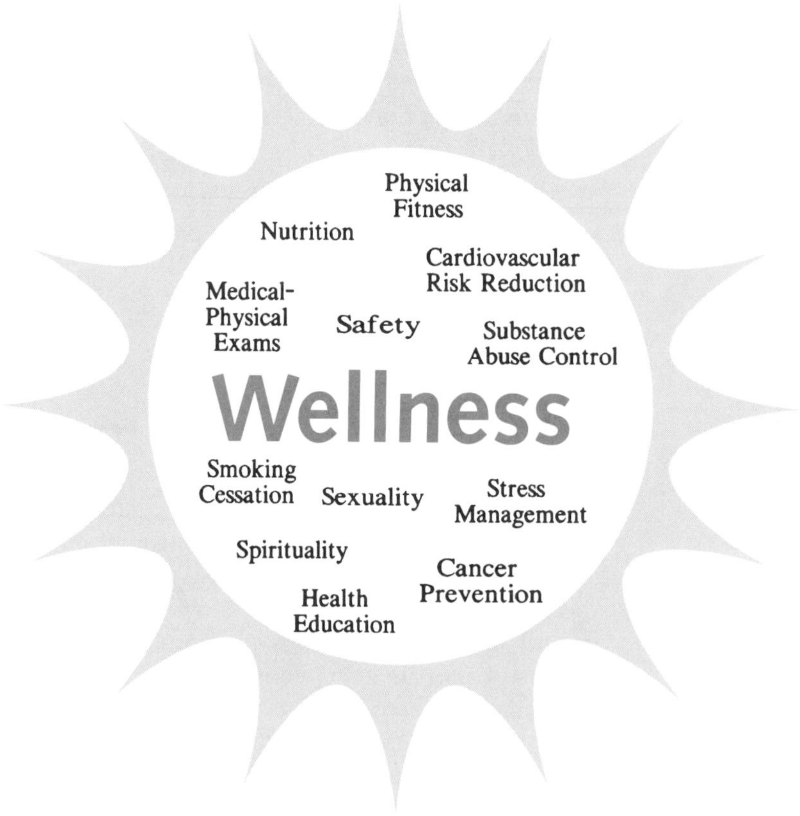

Wellness Components

asymptomatic state produced by a negative health behavior that may lead to disease.

Consequently, our biggest challenge at the end of this century is to teach people how to take control of their personal health habits by engaging in positive lifestyle activities. To help you determine how your lifestyle habits are contributing to your health, the National Health Information Clearinghouse developed a simple "healthstyle self-test." This test is contained in Appendix F.

Researchers also point out seven simple lifestyle habits that can significantly increase longevity:

1. Participate in a lifetime exercise program.

2. Sleep 7 to 8 hours each night.

3. Eat breakfast every day.

4. Do not eat between meals.

5. Eat less sweets and fat.

6. Maintain recommended body weight.

7. Avoid chemical dependency (includes drinking only moderate amounts of alcohol or none at all, not smoking cigarettes, and refraining from all other hard drug use).

MAJOR HEALTH PROBLEMS IN THE UNITED STATES

Approximately 70% of all deaths in the United States are caused by cardiovascular disease and cancer. Close to 80% of these deaths could be prevented by a healthy lifestyle program. Accidents are the third leading cause of death. Although not all accidents are preventable, many are. Fatal accidents frequently are related to drug abuse and to not using seat belts. The fourth leading cause of death, chronic and obstructive pulmonary disease, is attributed largely to tobacco use.

CARDIOVASCULAR DISEASE

The most prevalent degenerative diseases in the United States are those of the cardiovascular system. *Nearly half of all deaths in this country are attributed to heart and blood vessel disease.* Some examples of cardiovascular diseases are coronary heart disease, peripheral vascular disease, congenital heart disease, rheumatic heart disease, atherosclerosis, strokes, high blood pressure, and congestive heart failure. Table 6.1 provides the estimated prevalence and number of deaths caused by the major types of cardiovascular disease in 1989.

TABLE 6.1

Estimated Prevalence and Number of Deaths from Cardiovascular Disease: 1989

	Prevalence	Deaths
Major forms of cardiovascular diseases*	69,080,000	944,688
Coronary heart disease	6,160,000	**
Heart attack	1,500,000	500,000
Stroke	2,980,000	147,470
High blood pressure	62,770,000	31,630
Rheumatic heart disease	1,310,000	6,000

*Includes people with one or more forms of cardiovascular disease.
**Number of deaths included under heart attack.

Sources: American Heart Association and National Center for Health Statistics (U.S. Public Health Service, Department of Health and Human Services).

According to the American Heart Association, the estimated cost of heart and blood vessel disease in 1991 exceeded $101 billion. Heart attacks alone cost American industry approximately 132 million workdays annually, including $15 billion in lost productivity because of physical and emotional disability.

More than 1.5 million people have heart attacks each year, and over half a million of them die as a result. About half the time, the first symptom of coronary heart disease is the heart attack itself, and 40% of the people who have a first heart attack die within the first 24 hours. In one of every five cardiovascular deaths, sudden death is the initial symptom. About half of those who die are men in their most productive years — between the ages of 40 and 65.

Although heart and blood vessel disease is still the number one health problem in the United States, the incidence has declined by 36% in the last two decades. The main reason for this dramatic decrease is health education. More people are now aware of the risk factors for cardiovascular disease and are changing their lifestyle to lower their potential risk for this disease.

The major form of cardiovascular disease is coronary heart disease (CHD). The heart and the coronary arteries are illustrated in Figure 6.2. CHD is *a condition in which the arteries that supply the heart muscle with oxygen and nutrients are narrowed by fatty deposits such as cholesterol and triglycerides.* Narrowing of the coronary arteries diminishes the blood supply to the heart muscle, which can precipitate a heart attack. CHD is the single leading cause of death in the United States, accounting for approximately a third of all deaths and more than half of all cardiovascular deaths.

The leading risk factors contributing to the development of CHD are listed in Figure 6.3. An important concept in CHD risk management is that, with the exception of age, family history of heart disease, and certain electrocardiogram abnormalities, all the other risk factors are preventable and reversible, and individuals can control them by modifying

FIGURE 6.2

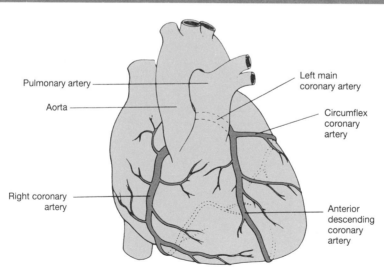

Pulmonary artery

Aorta

Right coronary artery

Left main coronary artery

Circumflex coronary artery

Anterior descending coronary artery

The heart and its blood vessels (coronary arteries).

FIGURE 6.3

Leading Risk Factors for Coronary Heart Disease

- Low HDL-cholesterol
- Elevated LDL-cholesterol
- Smoking
- Low cardiovascular fitness
- High blood pressure
- Elevated triglycerides
- High body fat
- Diabetes
- Abnormal electrocardiogram (ECG)
- Tension and stress
- Personal and family history
- Age

FIGURE 6.4

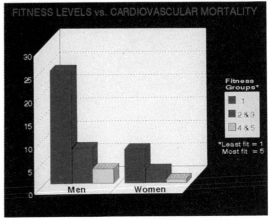

Relationship Between Fitness Levels and Cardio-vascular Mortality (age-adjusted death rates per 10,000 person-years of follow-up, 1970-1985).

Based on data from Blair, S. N., H. W. Kohl III, R. S. Paffenbarger, Jr., D. G. Clark, K. H. Cooper, and L. W. Gibbons. "Physical Fitness and All-Cause Mortality: A Prospective Study of Healthy Men and Women." JAMA 262:2395-2401, 1989.

their lifestyle. To aid in implementing a life-time risk reduction program, the guidelines described next should be implemented.

Cardiovascular Endurance

Improving cardiovascular endurance through aerobic exercise has perhaps the greatest impact in overall heart disease risk reduction. In this day and age, we cannot afford not to exercise. According to Dr. Kenneth H. Cooper, pioneer of the aerobic movement in the United States, "The evidence of the benefits of aerobic exercise in the reduction of heart disease is far too impressive to be ignored."

The guidelines for implementing an aerobic exercise program are discussed thoroughly in Chapter 3. Although these guidelines are ideal for proper cardiovascular fitness development, even smaller amounts of aerobic exercise can considerably reduce cardiovascular risk.

As shown in Figure 6.4, work conducted at the Aerobics Research Institute in Dallas demonstrated a large reduction in cardiovascular mortality when people abandon a sedentary lifestyle (group 1 in Figure 6.4) and initiate a

moderate aerobic exercise program (groups 2 and 3). The researchers recommended a minimum exercise dose for adults to achieve moderate fitness. The minimum exercise dose is presented in Figure 6.5.

Blood Pressure

Blood pressure should be checked regularly, regardless of whether it is or is not elevated. The pressure is measured in milliliters of mercury (mmHg) and usually expressed in two numbers. The higher number reflects the *systolic pressure or the pressure exerted during the forceful contraction of the heart. The lower value or diastolic pressure is taken during the heart's relaxation phase,* when no blood is being ejected.

Ideal blood pressure is 120/80 or below. The American Heart Association considers all blood pressures over 140/90 as *hypertension.*

FIGURE 6.5

Minimum Exercise Dose for Moderate Fitness

	Activity	Distance (miles)	Time (min.)	Frequency (days/week)
Women				
Program I:	Walking	3 or more	30 or less	3 or more
Program II:	Walking	2	30–40	5-6
Men				
Program I:	Walking	2	27 or less	3 or more
Program II:	Walking	2	30–40	6–7

From Blair, S.N. Fitness and Mortality. Dallas: Aerobics Research Center Longitudinal Study, 1991.

Regular aerobic exercise, weight control, a low-salt, low-fat diet, smoking cessation, and stress management are the keys to blood pressure control.

Body Composition

As discussed in Chapters 2 and 3, body composition is the ratio of lean body weight to fat weight. If too much fat is accumulated, the person is considered to be obese. *Obesity has long been recognized as a risk factor for coronary heart disease.* Maintaining recommended body weight (fat percent) is essential in any cardiovascular risk reduction program. Guidelines for a weight control program are presented in Chapter 5.

Blood Lipids

The term *blood lipids* (fats) is used mainly in reference to cholesterol and triglycerides. If you have never had a blood lipid test, it is highly recommended. The blood test should include total cholesterol, high-density lipoprotein cholesterol (HDL-cholesterol), low-density lipoprotein cholesterol (LDL-cholesterol), and triglycerides. A significant elevation in blood lipids has been clearly linked to heart and blood vessel disease.

A poor blood lipid profile is thought to be the most important predisposing factor in the development of CHD, accounting for almost half of all cases. The general recommendation by the National Cholesterol Education Program (NCEP) is to keep total cholesterol levels below 200 mg/dl (see Table 6.2). Cholesterol levels between 200 and 239 mg/dl are borderline high, and levels of 240 mg/dl and above indicate high risk for disease.

Many preventive medicine practitioners, however, recommend that total cholesterol should range between 160 and 180 mg/dl. For children the level should always be below 170 mg/dl. In the Framingham Heart Study, a 40-year ongoing project in the community of Framingham, Massachusetts, not a single individual with a total cholesterol level of 150 mg/dl or lower has had a heart attack.

Perhaps even more significant is the way in which cholesterol is carried in the bloodstream. Cholesterol is transported primarily by HDL and LDL molecules. The high-density molecules tend to attract cholesterol, which is carried to the liver to be metabolized and excreted. HDLs act as "scavengers," removing

TABLE 6.2

Standards for Blood Lipids

Total Cholesterol	≤200 mg/dl	Desirable
	201-239 mg/dl	Borderline high
	≥240 mg/dl	High risk
LDL-Cholesterol	≤130 mg/dl	Desirable
	131-159 mg/dl	Borderline high
	≥160 mg/dl	High risk
HDL-Cholesterol	≥45 mg/dl	Desirable
	36-44 mg/dl	Moderate risk
	≤35 mg/dl	High risk
Triglycerides	≤250 mg/dl	Desirable
	251-499 mg/dl	Borderline high
	≥500 mg/dl	High risk

cholesterol from the body and preventing plaque from forming in the arteries.

LDL-cholesterol, on the other hand, tends to release cholesterol, which then may penetrate the lining of the arteries and speed up the process of atherosclerosis. The NCEP guidelines state that an LDL-cholesterol value below 130 mg/dl is desirable, between 130 and 159 mg/dl is borderline-high, and 160 mg/dl and above is high risk for cardiovascular disease.

The more HDL-cholesterol the better. *HDL-cholesterol is the "good cholesterol"* and offers some protection against heart disease. In fact, new evidence suggests that low levels of HDL-cholesterol could be the best predictor of CHD and may be more significant than the total value. Substantial research supports the evidence that a low level of HDL-cholesterol has the strongest relationship to CHD at all levels of total cholesterol, including levels below 200 mg/dl.

Researchers at the 1988 annual American Heart Association meeting found that people with low total cholesterol (less than 200 mg/dl) and also low HDL-cholesterol (under 40 mg/dl) may have three times greater heart disease risk than those with high cholesterol but with good HDL-cholesterol levels. The recommended HDL-cholesterol values to minimize the risk for CHD are 45 mg/dl or higher.

Increasing the HDL-cholesterol improves the cholesterol profile and decreases the risk for CHD. Habitual aerobic exercise, weight loss, and quitting smoking have all been shown to raise HDL-cholesterol. Beta-carotene and drug therapy also promote higher HDL-cholesterol levels.

If LDL-cholesterol is higher than ideal, it can be lowered by losing body fat, taking medication, and manipulating the diet. A diet low in fat, saturated fat, and cholesterol , and high in fiber is recommended to decrease LDL-cholesterol. The NCEP recommends replacing saturated fat with monounsaturated fat (for example, olive, canola, peanut, and sesame oils), because the latter does not cause a reduction in HDL-cholesterol.

Many experts believe that to have a significant effect in lowering LDL-cholesterol, total fat consumption must be significantly lower than the current 30% of total daily caloric intake guideline. Saturated fat consumption should be 10% or less of the total daily caloric intake, and the average cholesterol consumption should be much lower than 300 mg per day.

Research studies on the effects of a 30%-fat diet have shown that it has little or no effect in lowering cholesterol and that CHD actually continues to progress in people who have the disease. The good news comes from a 1991 study published in the Archives of Internal Medicine which reported that the men and women in the study lowered their cholesterol by an average of 23% in only three weeks following a 10% or less fat-calorie-diet combined with a regular aerobic exercise program, primarily walking. In this diet, cholesterol intake was limited to less than 25 mg/day. The author of the study concluded that the exact percent fat guideline (10 or 15) is unknown (it also varies from individual to individual), but that 30% total fat calories is definitely too high a level when attempting to decrease cholesterol.

A daily 10%-total-fat-diet requires that the person limit fat intake to an absolute minimum. Some health care professionals contend that a diet like this is difficult to follow indefinitely. People with high cholesterol levels, however, may not need to follow that diet indefinitely but should adopt the 10%-fat-diet while attempting to lower cholesterol. Thereafter, eating a 30%-fat-diet may be adequate to maintain recommended cholesterol levels (1991 national data indicate that current fat consumption in the United States averages 37% of total calories — see Figure 5.2 in Chapter 5).

As a rule of thumb, the following dietary guidelines are recommended to lower LDL-cholesterol levels:

1. Egg consumption of fewer than three eggs per week.

2. Red meats (3 ounce per serving) fewer than three times per week, and no organ meats (such as liver and kidneys).

3. No commercially baked foods.

4. Low-fat milk (1% or less fat, preferably) and low-fat dairy products.

5. No coconut oil, palm oil, or cocoa butter.

6. Fish, especially those high in Omega-3 fatty acids (fresh or frozen mackerel, herring, tuna, salmon, and lake trout) twice a week.

7. Attainment of recommended body weight.

The antioxidant effect of Vitamins C and E and beta-carotene can also reduce the risk for

CHD. New information suggests that a single unstable free radical (oxygen compounds produced in normal metabolism) can damage LDL particles. Vitamin C seems to inactivate free radicals, and vitamin E protects LDL from oxidation. Beta-carotene not only absorbs free radicals, keeping them from causing damage, but it also seems to increase HDL levels.

Triglycerides also are known as free fatty acids. In combination with cholesterol, they speed up the formation of plaque. Triglycerides are carried in the bloodstream mainly by very low-density lipoproteins (VLDLs) and chylomicrons. These fatty acids are found in poultry skin, lunch meats, and shellfish, but they are manufactured mainly in the liver, from refined sugars, starches, and alcohol. High intake of alcohol and sugars (honey included) significantly raises triglyceride levels. The level can be lowered by cutting down on these foods along with reducing weight (if overweight) and doing aerobic exercise. An ideal blood triglyceride level is 100 mg/dl or lower, although up to 250 mg/dl is still considered acceptable (see Table 6.2).

Diabetes

Diabetes mellitus is a condition in which the blood glucose is unable to enter the cells because the pancreas either totally stops producing insulin or does not produce enough to meet the body's needs. *The incidence of cardiovascular disease and death in the diabetic population is quite high.* People with chronically elevated blood glucose levels also may have problems in metabolizing fats, which can make them more susceptible to atherosclerosis, increase the risk for coronary disease, and lead to other conditions such as vision loss and kidney damage.

Although there is a genetic predisposition to diabetes, adult-onset or Type II diabetes is closely related to overeating, obesity, and lack of physical activity. In most cases, this condition can be corrected through a special diet, a weight-loss program, and a regular exercise program. A diet high in water-soluble fibers (found in fruits, vegetables, oats, and beans) is helpful in treating diabetes. A simple aerobic exercise program (walking, cycling, or swimming four to five times per week) is often prescribed because it increases the body's sensitivity to insulin. Individuals who have high blood glucose levels should consult a physician to decide on the best treatment.

Electrocardiograms (ECG)

The ECG provides a record of the electrical impulses that stimulate the heart to contract. ECGs are taken at rest, during the stress of exercise (Figure 2.2 in Chapter 2), and during recovery. An exercise ECG also is known as a graded exercise stress test or a maximal exercise tolerance test. Similar to a high-speed road test on a car, *a stress ECG reveals the heart's tolerance to high-intensity exercise.* Based on the findings, ECGs may be interpreted as normal, equivocal, or abnormal.

A stress ECG frequently is used to diagnose coronary heart disease. It also is administered to determine cardiovascular fitness levels, to screen individuals for preventive and cardiac rehabilitation programs, to detect abnormal blood pressure response during exercise, and to establish actual or functional maximal heart rate for exercise prescription purposes.

Not every adult who wishes to start or continue in an exercise program needs a stress ECG. The following guidelines can help you determine when this type of test should be conducted:

1. Men over age 40 and women over age 50.

2. A total cholesterol level above 200 mg/dl, or an HDL-cholesterol level below 35 mg/dl.

3. Hypertensive and diabetic patients.

4. Cigarette smokers.

5. Individuals with a family history of CHD, syncope, or sudden death before age 60.

6. People with an abnormal resting ECG.

7. All individuals with symptoms of chest discomfort, dysrhythmias, syncope, or chronotropic incompetence (a heart rate that increases slowly during exercise and never reaches maximum).

Smoking

More than 47 million adults and 3.5 million adolescents in the United States smoke. *Cigarette smoking is the single largest preventable cause of illness and premature death in the United States.* When considering all related deaths, tobacco is responsible for 350,000 unnecessary deaths per year. About 50,000 of those who die are nonsmokers who were exposed to second-hand smoke. Smoking has been linked to cardiovascular disease, cancer, bronchitis, emphysema, and peptic ulcers.

In relation to coronary disease, not only does smoking speed up the process of atherosclerosis, but it produces a threefold increase in the risk of sudden death following a myocardial infarction. Smoking increases the heart rate, raises blood pressure, and irritates the heart, which can trigger fatal cardiac arrhythmias (irregular heart rhythms). As far as the extra load on the heart is concerned, giving up one pack of cigarettes per day is the equivalent of losing between 50 and 75 pounds of excess body fat! Another harmful effect is a decrease in HDL-cholesterol, the "good" type that helps control blood lipids.

Pipe and cigar smoking and chewing tobacco also increase the risk for heart disease. Even if no smoke is inhaled, toxic substances are absorbed through the membranes of the mouth and end up in the bloodstream. Individuals who use tobacco in any of these three forms also have a much greater risk for cancer of the oral cavity.

Cigarette smoking, a poor cholesterol profile, low fitness, and high blood pressure are the four major risk factors for coronary disease. Nonetheless, the risk for both cardiovascular disease and cancer starts to decrease the moment you quit smoking. The risk approaches that of a lifetime non-smoker 10 and 15 years, respectively, after cessation.

Quitting cigarette smoking is no easy task. Surveys indicate that nine of ten smokers want to quit. Only about 20% of smokers who try to quit for the first time succeed each year. The addictive properties of nicotine and smoke make quitting very difficult. Smokers experience physical and psychological withdrawal symptoms when they stop smoking. Even though giving up smoking can be extremely hard, cessation is by no means impossible.

The most important factor in quitting cigarette smoking is the person's sincere desire to do so. More than 95% of the successful ex-smokers have been able to quit on their own, either by quitting cold turkey or by using self-help kits available from organizations such as the American Cancer Society, the American Heart Association, and the American Lung Association. Only 3% of ex-smokers quit as a result of formal cessation programs. A six-step plan to help people stop smoking is contained in Figure 6.6.

Tension and Stress

Tension and stress have become a normal part of life. Everyone has to deal daily with goals, deadlines, responsibilities, pressures. Almost everything in life (whether positive or negative) is a source of stress. The stressor itself is not what creates the health hazard but, rather, the individual's response to it. *Individuals who are under a lot of stress and cannot relax place a constant low-level strain on the cardiovascular system that could manifest itself in the form of heart disease.*

Learning to live and get ahead today is virtually impossible without practicing adequate stress management techniques. Perhaps the three most common stress management techniques available are physical exercise, progressive muscle relaxation, and breathing techniques. These techniques are discussed next.

Physical exercise is one of the simplest tools to control stress. Exercise and fitness are thought to reduce the intensity of the stress response and the recovery time from a stressful event. The value of exercise in reducing stress is related to several factors, the main one being less muscular tension.

For example, a person may be distressed because he or she has a miserable day at work and the job requires 8 hours of work in a smoke-filled room with an intolerable boss. To make matters worse, it is late and on the way home the car in front is going much slower than the speed limit. The body's "fight or flight" mechanism is activated, heart rate and blood pressure shoot up, breathing quickens and deepens, muscles tense up, and all systems say "go." But no action can be initiated, or stress dissipated, because you just cannot hit your boss or the car in front of you. A person surely could take action, however, by "hitting" the tennis ball, the weights, the swimming pool, or the jogging trail. By engaging in physical activity, a person is able to reduce the muscular tension and eliminate the physiological changes that triggered the fight or flight mechanism.

Progressive muscle relaxation is one of the most popular procedures used to dissipate stress. This technique enables individuals to relearn the sensation of deep relaxation. It

FIGURE 6.6

Six-Step Smoking Cessation Approach

The following six-step plan has been developed as a guide to help you quit smoking. The total program should be completed in four weeks or less. Steps one through four should take no longer than two weeks. A maximum of two additional weeks are allowed for the rest of the program.

Step One. The first step in breaking the habit is to decide positively that you want to quit. Now prepare a list of the reasons why you smoke and why you want to quit.

Step Two. Initiate a personal diet and exercise program. Exercise and decreased body weight cause a greater awareness of healthy living and increase motivation for giving up cigarettes.

Step Three. Decide on the approach that you will use to stop smoking. You may quit cold turkey or gradually decrease the number of cigarettes smoked daily. Many people have found that quitting cold turkey is the easiest way to do it. While it may not work the first time, after several attempts, all of a sudden smokers are able to overcome the habit without too much difficulty. Tapering off cigarettes can be done in several ways. You may start by eliminating cigarettes that you do not necessarily need, you can switch to a brand lower in nicotine and/or tar every couple of days, you can smoke less off each cigarette, or you can simply decrease the total number of cigarettes smoked each day.

Step Four. Set the target date for quitting. In setting the target date, choosing a special date may add a little extra incentive. An upcoming birthday, anniversary, vacation, graduation, family reunion, etc., are all examples of good dates to free yourself from smoking.

Step Five. Stock up on low-calorie foods — carrots, broccoli, cauliflower, celery, popcorn (butter and salt free), fruits, sunflower seeds (in the shell), sugarless gum, and plenty of water. Keep such food handy on the day you stop and the first few days following cessation. Replace such food for cigarettes when you want one.

Step Six. This is the day that you will quit smoking. On this day and the first few days thereafter, do not keep cigarettes handy. Stay away from friends and events that trigger your desire to smoke. You should drink large amounts of water, fruit juices, and eat low calorie foods. An important factor in breaking the habit is to replace the old behavior with new behavior. You will need to replace smoking time with new positive substitutes that will make smoking difficult or impossible. When you desire a cigarette, take a few deep breaths and then occupy yourself by doing a number of things such as talking to someone else, washing your hands, brushing your teeth, eating a healthy snack, chewing on a straw, doing dishes, playing sports, going for a walk or bike ride, going swimming, and so on.

If you have been successful and stopped smoking, remember that there are a lot of events that can still trigger your urge to smoke. When confronted with such events, people rationalize and think, "One will not hurt." It will not work! Before you know, you will be back to the regular nasty habit. Therefore, be prepared to take action in those situations. Find adequate substitutes for smoking. Remind yourself of how difficult it has been and how long it has taken you to get to this point. Keep in mind that it will only get easier rather than worse as time goes on.

involves contraction and relaxation of muscle groups throughout the body. Since chronic stress leads to high muscular tension, being closely aware of how it feels to progressively tighten and relax the muscles will release the tension on the muscles and teach the body to relax at will. Being aware of the tension felt during the exercises also helps the person to be more alert to signs of distress, since similar feelings are experienced in stressful situations. In everyday life, these feelings can then be used as a cue to implement relaxation exercises.

Relaxation exercises should be done in a quiet, warm, well-ventilated room. The recommended exercises and the length of the routine vary from one expert to the next. Most important, the person must pay attention to the sensation felt each time the muscles are tensed and relaxed. The exercises should cover all muscle groups. An example of a sequence of progressive muscle relaxation exercises is given in Figure 6.7. The instructions outlined for these exercises can be read to the person, memorized, or tape-recorded. At least twenty minutes should be set aside to perform the entire sequence. Doing them any faster will defeat their purpose. Ideally, a person should repeat the sequence twice a day.

If time is a factor and an individual is not able to go through the entire sequence, only the exercises specific to the area where muscle tension is felt may be done. Performing just a few exercises is better than doing none at all. Of course, completing the whole sequence gives the best results.

Breathing exercises also can serve as an antidote to stress. These have been done for centuries in the Orient and India to improve mental, physical, and emotional stamina. The person concentrates on "breathing away" the tension and inhaling fresh air to the entire body. Breathing exercises can be learned in only a few minutes and require considerably less time than other forms of stress management. An example of these exercises is given in Figure 6.8.

Personal and Family History

Individuals who have a family history of, or already have suffered from, cardiovascular problems are at higher risk than those who have never had a problem. People with this sort of history should be strongly encouraged to keep the other risk factors as low as possible. Because most risk factors are reversible, this practice significantly decreases the risk for future problems.

Age

Age is a risk factor because of the greater incidence of heart disease in older people. This tendency may be induced partly by other factors stemming from changes in lifestyle as we get older (less physical activity, poor nutrition, obesity, and so on).

Young people should not think that heart disease will not affect them. The process begins early in life. It was clearly shown in American soldiers who died during the Korean and Vietnam conflicts. Autopsies conducted on soldiers killed at 22 years of age and younger revealed that approximately 70% had early stages of atherosclerosis. Other studies found elevated blood cholesterol levels in children as young as 10 years old.

Even though the aging process cannot be stopped, it certainly can be slowed down. Physiological versus chronological age is an important concept in preventing disease. Some individuals in their 60s or older have the body of a 20-year-old. And 20-year-olds often are in such poor condition and health that they almost seem to have the body of a 60-year-old. Risk factor management and positive lifestyle habits are the best ways to slow down the natural aging process.

FIGURE 6.7

Progressive Muscle Relaxation Sequence

Stretch out comfortably on the floor, face up, with a pillow under the knees, and assume a passive attitude, allowing the body to relax as much as possible. Contracts each muscle group in sequence, taking care to avoid any strain. Muscle tightening should be limited to about 70 percent of the total possible tension, to prevent cramping or injury to the muscle itself. Paying attention to the sensation of tensing up and relaxing is crucial to produce the relaxation effects. Each contraction is held for about five seconds, and then the muscles should be allowed to go totally limp. Sufficient time should be allowed for contraction and relaxation before the next instruction.

1. Point your feet, curling the toes downward, and study the tension in the arches and the top of the feet. Hold it and continue to note the tension, then relax. Repeat a second time.

2. Flex the feet upward toward the face and note the tension in your feet and calves. Hold it, and relax. Repeat again.

3. Push your heels down against the floor as if burying them in the sand. Hold it and note the tension on the back of the thigh; relax. Repeat one more time.

4. Contract the right thigh by straightening the leg, gently raising the leg off the floor. Hold it and study the tension; relax. Repeat with the left leg; hold and relax. Repeat both legs again.

5. Tense the buttocks by raising your hips ever so slightly off the floor. Hold it and note the tension, and relax. Repeat again.

6. Contract the abdominal muscles. Hold them tight and note the tension; relax. Repeat one more time.

7. Suck in your stomach — try to make it reach your spine. Flatten your lower back to the floor; hold it and feel the tension in the stomach and lower back; relax. Repeat again.

8. Take a deep breath and hold it, then exhale. Repeat again. Note your breathing becoming slower and more relaxed.

9. Place your arms on the side of your body and clench both fists. Hold it, study the tension, and relax.

10. Flex the elbow by bringing both hands to the shoulders. Hold it tight and study the tension in the biceps; relax. Repeat again.

11. Place your arms flat on the floor, palms up, and push the forearm hard against the floor. Note the tension on the triceps; hold it, and relax. Repeat the exercise.

12. Shrug your shoulders, raising them as high as possible. Hold it and note the tension; relax. Repeat again.

13. Gently push your head backward; note the tension in the back of the neck. Hold it, relax. Repeat one more time.

14. Gently bring the head against the chest, push forward, hold, and note the tension in the neck. Relax. Repeat a second time.

15. Press your tongue toward the roof of your mouth. Hold it, study the tension; relax. Repeat again.

16. Press your teeth together. Hold it and study the tension; relax. Repeat again.

17. Close your eyes tightly. Hold them closed and note the tension. Relax, leaving your eyes closed. Repeat again.

18. Wrinkle your forehead. Note the tension; hold it, and relax. Repeat one more time.

FIGURE 6.8

Breathing Exercises for Stress Management

A quiet, pleasant, and well-ventilated room should be used to perform breathing exercises. Any of the three exercises listed below may be performed whenever tension is felt due to stress.

Deep breathing: Lie with your back flat against the floor, place a pillow under your knees, feet slightly separated, with toes pointing outward (the exercise may also be conducted sitting up in a chair or standing straight up). Place one hand on your abdomen and the other one on your chest. Slowly breathe in and out so that the hand on your abdomen rises when you inhale and falls as you exhale. The hand on the chest should not move much at all. Repeat the exercise about ten times. Next, scan your body for tension, and compare your present tension with that felt at the beginning of the exercise. Repeat the entire process once or twice more.

Sighing: Using the abdominal breathing technique, breathe in through your nose to a specific count (i.e., 4, 5, 6, etc.). Now exhale through pursed lips to double the intake count (i.e., 8, 10, 12, etc.). Repeat the exercise eight to ten times whenever you feel tense.

Complete natural breathing: Sit in an upright position or stand straight up. Breathe through your nose and gradually fill up your lungs from the bottom up. Hold your breath for several seconds. Now exhale slowly by allowing complete relaxation of the chest and abdomen. Repeat the exercise eight to ten times.

CANCER

Cancer is defined as an uncontrolled growth and spread of abnormal cells in the body, forming a mass of tissue called a tumor, which can be either benign or malignant. A malignant tumor is a "cancer." Cancer cells grow for no reason and multiply, destroying normal tissue. If the spread of cells is not controlled, death ensues. More than 22% of all deaths in the United States are from cancer. An estimated one million new cases are reported, and about half a million people die each year from cancer.

As with cardiovascular disease, cancer is largely preventable. *As much as 80% of all human cancers is related to lifestyle or environmental factors* (including diet, tobacco use, excessive use of alcohol, sexual and reproductive history, and exposure to occupational hazards). Most of these cancers could be prevented through positive life habits.

Equally important is the fact that cancer is now viewed as the most curable of all chronic diseases. More than half of all cancers are curable. In 1992, at least 7 million Americans with a history of cancer were alive, close to 3 million of whom were considered cured.

The most effective way to protect against cancer is by changing negative longstanding habits and behaviors. The following general recommendations have been issued in regard to cancer prevention (also see Figure 6.9):

Dietary Changes

According to the National Cancer Institute, about 40 and 60% of all cancers in men and women, respectively, are dietary related. A

FIGURE 6.9

ARE YOU TAKING CONTROL?

Today, scientists think most cancers may be related to lifestyle and environment — what you eat, drink, if you smoke and where you work and play. So the good news is you can help reduce your own cancer risk by taking control of things in your daily life.

10 Steps To A Healthier Life and Reduced Cancer Risk

1. **Are you eating more cabbage-family vegetables?**
    They include broccoli, cauliflower, brussels sprouts, all cabbages and kale.

2. **Are high-fiber foods included in your diet?**
    Fiber occurs in whole grains, fruits and vegetables including peaches, strawberries, potatoes, spinach, tomatoes, wheat and bran cereals, rice, popcorn and whole-wheat bread.

3. **Do you choose foods with Vitamin A?**
    Fresh foods with beta-carotene like carrots, peaches, apricots, squash and broccoli are the best source, not vitamin pills.

4. **Is Vitamin C included in your diet?**
    You'll find it naturally in lots of fresh fruits and vegetables like grapefruit, cantaloupe, oranges, strawberries, red and green peppers, broccoli and tomatoes.

5. **Do you exercise and monitor calorie intake to avoid weight gain?**
    Walking is ideal exercise for many people.

6. **Are you cutting overall fat intake?**
    This is done by eating lean meat, fish, skinned poultry and low-fat dairy products.

7. **Do you limit salt-cured, smoked, nitrite-cured foods?**
    Choose bacon, ham, hot dogs or salt-cured fish only occasionally if you like them a lot.

8. **If you smoke, have you tried quitting?**

9. **If you drink alcohol, are you moderate in your intake?**

10. **Do you respect the sun's rays?**
    Protect yourself with sunscreen — at least #15, wear long sleeves and a hat, especially during midday hours — 11 a.m. to 3 p.m.

If you answer yes to most of these questions, **Congratulations**. You are taking control of simple lifestyle factors that will help you feel better and reduce your cancer risk.

*Courtesy of the Texas Division of the American Cancer Society.

Cancer prevention questionnaire.

recommended cancer prevention diet should be low in fat and high in fiber, and contain vitamins A and C from natural sources. Protein intake should be within the RDA guidelines. The diet should include cruciferous vegetables (plants that produce cross-shaped leaves). Alcohol should be consumed in moderation, and obesity should be avoided.

High fat intake has been linked primarily to breast, colon, and prostate cancers. Low fiber intake seems to increase the risk of colon cancer. Foods high in vitamin A and C may deter larynx, esophagus, and lung cancers. Salt-cured, smoked, and nitrite-cured foods have been associated with cancer of the esophagus and stomach. Vitamin C seems to discourage the formation of nitrosamines (cancer-causing substances formed from eating cured meats).

Carrots, squash, sweet potatoes, and cruciferous vegetables (cauliflower, broccoli, cabbage, Brussels sprouts, and kohlrabi) seem to protect against cancer. These vegetables contain a lot of beta-carotene (a precursor to vitamin A) and vitamin C. Although the cancer-protecting mechanism of these vegetables is not known, researchers believe the antioxidant effect of these vitamins protects the body from oxygen free radicals.

Daily protein intake for many Americans is almost twice the amount the human body needs. Too much animal protein decreases blood enzymes that prevent precancerous cells from developing into tumors. Other research suggests that carcinogenic substances form on the skin or surface of the meat when grilled at high temperatures for a long time. Microwaving the meat for a couple of minutes before barbecuing decreases the risk, as long as the fluid the meat releases is discarded. Most potential carcinogens collect in this solution. Removing the skin before serving and cooking the meat at lower heat to a medium stage rather than well done also seems to decrease the risk.

Excessive alcohol consumption raises the risk for developing certain cancers, especially when it is combined with tobacco smoking or smokeless tobacco. In combination, these substances significantly increase the risk of mouth, larynx, throat, esophagus, and liver cancers. According to some research, the combined action of heavy use of alcohol and tobacco increases cancer of the oral cavity fifteen-fold.

Maintaining recommended body weight is also encouraged. Obesity has been associated with colon, rectum, breast, prostate, gallbladder, ovary, and uterine cancers.

Abstinence From Cigarette Smoking

The biggest carcinogenic exposure in the workplace today is cigarette smoke. It has been reported by the American Cancer Society that 83% of lung cancers and 30% of all cancers are linked to smoking. The use of smokeless tobacco also increases the risk of mouth, larynx, throat, and esophagus cancers. About 138,600 cancer deaths annually stem from tobacco use. The average life expectancy for a chronic smoker is 7 years less than for a nonsmoker.

Avoid Sun Exposure

Exposure to sunlight is a major factor in the development of skin cancer. *Nearly all of the 600,000 nonmelanoma skin cancer cases reported annually in the United States are related to sun exposure.* People should apply sunscreen lotion when the skin is going to be exposed to sunlight for extended periods. Tanning of the skin is the body's natural reaction to cell damage from excessive sun exposure. Even brief exposures add up to more risk of skin cancer and premature aging.

Sunscreen lotion should be applied about 30 minutes before lengthy exposure to the sun because the skin takes that long to absorb the protective ingredients. A sun protection factor (SPF) of at least 15 is recommended. SPF 15 means that the skin takes 15 times longer to burn than with no lotion. If you ordinarily get a mild sunburn after 20 minutes of noonday sun, an SPF 15 allows you to remain in the sun about 300 minutes before burning.

Avoid Estrogen, Radiation, and Occupational Hazards

Estrogen has been linked to endometrial cancer, but it can be taken safely under careful supervision by a physician. Although exposure to radiation increases the risk for cancer, the benefits of X-rays may outweigh the risk involved, and most medical facilities administer the lowest dose possible to keep the risk to a minimum. Occupational hazards, such as asbestos fibers, nickel and uranium dusts, chromium compounds, vinyl chloride, and bischlormethyl ether, increase cancer risk. Cigarette smoking magnifies the risk from occupational hazards.

Warning Signals For Cancer

Through early detection, many cancers can be controlled or cured. The real problem is the spreading of cancerous cells. Once that happens, it becomes difficult to wipe out the cancer. Therefore, effective prevention, or at least catching cancer when the possibility of cure is greatest, is crucial. Herein lies the importance of proper periodic screening for prevention and early detection.

Everyone should become familiar with the following seven warning signals for cancer and bring any of them to a physician's attention:

1. Change in bowel or bladder habits.

2. A sore that does not heal.

3. Unusual bleeding or discharge.

4. Thickening or lump in breast or elsewhere.

5. Indigestion or difficulty in swallowing.

6. Obvious change in wart or mole.

7. Nagging cough or hoarseness.

Scientific evidence and testing procedures for prevention and early detection of cancer do change. Studies continue to provide new information about cancer prevention and detection. The intent of cancer prevention programs is to educate and guide individuals toward a lifestyle that will help prevent cancer and enable early detection of malignancy. Treatment of cancer always should be left to specialized physicians and cancer clinics.

ACCIDENTS

Even though most people do not consider accidents a health problem, accidents are the third leading cause of death in the United States, affecting the total well-being of millions of Americans each year. Accident prevention and personal safety are also part of a health enhancement program aimed at achieving a higher quality of life. Proper nutrition, exercise, abstinence from cigarette smoking, and stress management are of little help if the person is involved in a disabling or fatal accident as a result of distraction, a single reckless decision, or not properly wearing safety seat belts.

Accidents do not just happen. We cause accidents, and we are victims of accidents. Although some factors in life, such as earthquakes, tornadoes, and airplane crashes, are completely beyond our control, *more often than not, personal safety and accident prevention are a matter of common sense.* Most accidents are precipitated by poor judgment and a confused mental state. Accidents frequently happen when we are upset, not paying attention, or abusing alcohol and other drugs.

Alcohol abuse is the number one cause of all accidents. Statistics clearly show that alcohol intoxication is the leading cause of fatal automobile accidents. Other drugs commonly abused in society alter feelings and perceptions, lead to mental confusion, and impair judgment and coordination, all of which greatly increase the risk for accidental morbidity and mortality.

CHRONIC OBSTRUCTIVE PULMONARY DISEASE

Chronic obstructive pulmonary disease (COPD) is a term encompassing diseases that limit air flow, such as chronic bronchitis, emphysema, and a reactive airway component similar to that of asthma. The incidence of COPD increases proportionately with cigarette smoking (or other forms of tobacco use) and exposure to certain types of industrial pollution. In the case of emphysema, genetic factors also may play a role.

SPIRITUAL WELL-BEING

The scientific association between spirituality and health is more difficult to establish than that of other lifestyle factors such as alcohol, smoking, physical inactivity, seat belt use, and so on. Even so, several research studies have reported positive relationships between health and spiritual well-being, emotional well-being, and life satisfaction. One study revealed a much higher rate of heart attacks in nonreligious people, compared to a sample of people who regularly attend church. Other studies suggest that religious support may act as a buffer against disease, that the social support encourages preventive health.

The National Interfaith Coalition on Aging has defined spiritual well-being as *an affirmation of life in a relationship with God, self, community, and environment that nurtures and celebrates wholeness* (Figure 6.10). This definition includes Christians and non-Christians alike and assumes that all people are spiritual in nature.

Wellness requires a balance among physical, mental, spiritual, emotional, and social components of well-being. The relationship between spirituality and wellness, therefore, is meaningful in the quest for a better quality of life. Religion has been a major part of cultures since the beginning of time. Although not everyone in the United States claims affiliation with a specific religion or denomination,

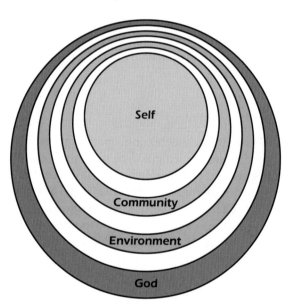

FIGURE 6.10

Spiritual

Self

Community

Environment

God

Well-being

Spiritual Well-being. An affirmation of life in a relationship with God, self, community, and environment that nurtures and celebrates wholeness.

current surveys indicate that 94% of the U.S. population believes in God or a universal spirit that functions as God. People, furthermore, believe to varying extents that (a) a relationship with God is meaningful; (b) God can grant help, guidance, and assistance in daily living; and (c) mortal existence has a purpose. If we accept any or all of these statements, attaining spirituality will affect one's happiness and well-being.

SUBSTANCE ABUSE CONTROL (CHEMICAL HEALTH)

Chemical dependency presently encompasses some of the most serious, self-destructive forms of addiction in our society, including alcohol, hard drugs, and cigarette smoking (the latter already has been discussed in this chapter). Other problems associated with substance abuse are drunken or impaired driving, mixing prescriptions, family difficulties, and drugs to improve athletic performance.

Alcohol represents one of the most significant health-related drug problems in the United States today. Estimates indicate that seven in ten adults, or more than 100 million Americans 18 years and older, are drinkers. Approximately 10 million of them will have a drinking problem, including alcoholism, in their lifetime. Another 3 million teenagers are thought to have a drinking problem.

Alcohol intake cuts down on peripheral vision, impairs the ability to see and hear, causes slower reactions, reduces concentration and motor performance (including swaying and poor judgment of distance and speed of moving objects), lessens fear, increases risk-taking behaviors, causes more frequent urination, and induces sleep. A single large dose of alcohol also may lower sexual function. One of the most unpleasant, dangerous, and life-threatening consequences of drinking is the synergistic action of alcohol when combined with other drugs, particularly central nervous system depressants.

Long-term manifestations of alcohol abuse can be serious and life-threatening. These conditions include cirrhosis of the liver (scarring of the liver, often fatal); greater risk for oral, esophageal, and liver cancer; cardiomyopathy (a disease that affects the heart muscle); high blood pressure; greater risk for strokes; inflammation of the esophagus, stomach, small intestine, and pancreas; stomach ulcers; sexual impotence; malnutrition; brain cell damage and consequent loss of memory; psychosis; depression; and hallucinations.

Approximately 60% of the world's production of illegal drugs is consumed in the United States. Each year Americans spend more than $100 billion on illegal drugs, surpassing the total dollars taken in from all crops produced by United States farmers. According to the U.S. Department of Education, today's drugs are stronger and more addictive, posing a greater risk than ever before. Drugs lead to physical and psychological dependence. If used regularly, they integrate into the body's chemistry, raising drug tolerance and forcing the person to constantly increase the dosage for similar results. Drug abuse leads not only to serious health problems; more than half of all adolescent suicides are drug-related.

Recognizing the hazards of chemical use, families, teams, and communities can assist each other in preventing problems, as well as help those who have problems with chemical use. Moreover, treating chemical dependency (including alcohol), is seldom accomplished without professional guidance and support. To secure the best available assistance, people in need should contact a physician or obtain a referral from a local mental health clinic (see Yellow Pages in the phone book.)

SEXUALLY TRANSMITTED DISEASES

Sexually transmitted diseases (STDs) have reached epidemic proportions in the United States. The American Social Health Association stated that *25% of all Americans will acquire at least one STD in their lifetime.* Of the more than twenty-five known STDs, some are still incurable. According to the Centers for Disease Control in Atlanta, more than 10 million people were newly infected with STDs in 1986, including 4.6 million cases of chlamydia, 1.8 million of gonorrhea, 1 million of genital warts, 500,000 of herpes, and 90,000 of syphilis. Attracting most of the attention because of its life-threatening potential were 15,000 new cases of AIDS (Acquired Immune Deficiency Syndrome).

AIDS is the most frightening of all STDs because it has no known cure and few have survived the disease. Anywhere from 1.5 to 4 million Americans are thought to carry the human immunodeficiency virus (HIV) that causes AIDS. By 1991, more than 100,000 people in the United States had died from AIDS. The HIV virus attacks cells, weakening the immune system. Although the number of carriers who will actually get AIDS is much debated, a third to a half will develop the disease. Even if a person doesn't develop AIDS, he or she can pass on the virus to others who could easily develop the disease (including pregnant women to their unborn babies). Unless a vaccine is found, it is projected that by the year 2000, more than 200,000 people will die from AIDS, making it the third leading cause of death, behind cardiovascular disease and cancer.

Many people believe that only certain "high-risk groups" of people are infected by the AIDS virus. This is untrue. Who you are has nothing to do with whether you are in danger of being infected with the AIDS virus. What matters is what you do.

High-risk individuals for AIDS are primarily (a) homosexual males with multiple sexual partners and (b) intravenous drug users, but health experts believe that in the future the disease may become just as common in heterosexuals. The virus is transmitted through blood and semen during sexual intercourse or by using hypodermic needles used previously by an infected individual. Anal intercourse, with or without a condom, is risky because the rectum is easily injured during anal intercourse.

AIDS cannot be contracted through everyday contact with people around you in school, in the workplace, at parties, child care centers, or stores. You will not get it by shaking hands with an infected person, from a toilet seat, from dishes or silverware used by an AIDS patient, by using a towel or clothes from a person with AIDS, or from donating blood. Furthermore, you will not get AIDS in a swimming pool, even if someone in the pool is infected with the AIDS virus. Students attending school with someone infected with the AIDS virus are not in danger from casual contact.

Once a person becomes infected with the AIDS virus, an incubation period ranging from a few months to 6 years ensues, during which time no symptoms appear. Eventually the virus weakens and incapacitates the immune system, leaving the person vulnerable to all types of infectious diseases and certain types of cancer. The AIDS virus itself doesn't kill. Rather, the ineffectiveness of the immune system in dealing with the various illnesses is what leads to death. Although several drugs are being tested to treat and slow down the disease process, AIDS has no known cure.

What about dating? Dating and getting to know other people are normal aspects of life. Dating, however, does not mean the same thing as having sex. Sexual intercourse as a part of dating can be risky, and one of the risks is AIDS. You can't tell if someone you are dating or would like to date has been exposed to the AIDS virus. The good news, though, is that as long as you avoid sexual activity and don't share drug needles, it doesn't matter whom you date.

The best way to prevent sexually transmitted diseases is through a mutually monogamous sexual relationship — sex with only one person who has sexual relationships only with you. Risky behaviors that significantly increase the chances of contracting sexually transmitted diseases, including AIDS, are:

■ multiple and/or anonymous sexual partners such as a pickup or prostitute.

■ anal sex with or without a condom.

■ vaginal or oral sex with someone who shoots drugs or engages in anal sex.

■ sex with someone you know has several sex partners.

■ unprotected sex (without a condom) with an infected person.

■ sexual contact (this includes open-mouthed or French kissing, as the AIDS virus may be present in saliva; note, however, that no evidence indicates AIDS has been transmitted in this way) with anyone who has symptoms

of AIDS or who is a member of a high-risk group for AIDS

■ sharing toothbrushes, razors, or other implements that could become contaminated with blood with anyone who is, or might be, infected with the AIDS virus.

IN CONCLUSION

Fitness and total well-being is a continual process. People need to put forth a constant, deliberate effort to achieve and maintain a higher quality of life. Implementing a program based on what you enjoy doing most, will make this journey easier and more fun along the way.

Your activities over the last few weeks or months may have helped you develop positive "addictions" that you should carry on throughout life. If you participate regularly and apply the principles explained in this book, you will truly experience a new quality of life. Once you reach the top, you will know there is no looking back. If you don't get there, you won't know what it's like. *Improving the quality and most likely the longevity of your life is now in your hands* (see Figure 6.11). It will require persistence and commitment, but *only you can take control of your lifestyle and thereby reap the benefits of wellness.*

FIGURE 6.11

A Wellness Way of Life

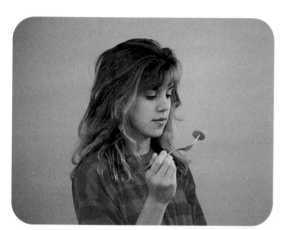

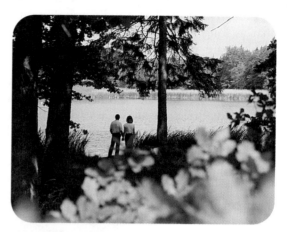

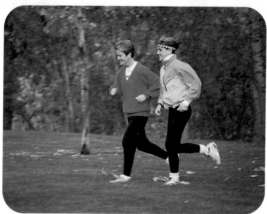

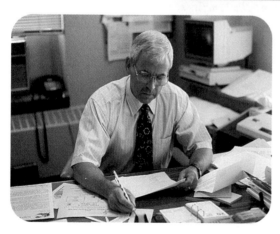

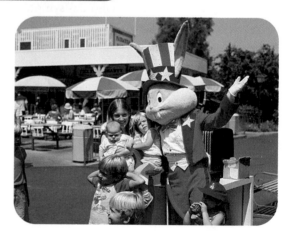

Relevant Questions and Answers Related to Fitness and Wellness

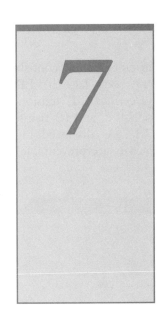

7

KEY CONCEPTS

- Cardiovascular disease
- Endorphines
- Concentric contraction
- Eccentric contraction
- Shin-splints
- Amenorrhea
- Dysmenorrhea
- Osteoporosis
- Kilocalorie
- Calorie

OBJECTIVES

- Clarify misconceptions related to physical fitness and wellness.

Some of the most frequently asked questions regarding various aspects of physical fitness and wellness are addressed in this chapter. The answers will further clarify concepts discussed throughout the book, as well as put to rest several myths that misinform fitness and wellness participants.

SAFETY OF EXERCISE PARTICIPATION AND INJURY PREVENTION

■ *Can aerobic exercise make a person immune to heart and blood vessel disease?*

Scientific evidence clearly indicates that aerobically fit individuals have a much lower incidence of cardiovascular disease. A regular aerobic exercise program by itself, however, is not an absolute guarantee against diseases of the heart and blood vessels. Several factors increase a person's risk for cardiovascular disease.

Though physical inactivity is one of the most significant risk factors, studies have documented that multiple interrelations usually exist between these risk factors. Physical inactivity, for instance, often contributes to an increase in (a) body fat, (b) LDL-cholesterol, (c) triglycerides, (d) tension and stress, (e) blood pressure, and (f) risk for diabetes (see Figure 7.1). As discussed in Chapter 6, most risk factors are preventable and reversible. Overall risk factor management is the best guideline to minimize the risk for cardiovascular disease. Research also indicates, however, that the odds of surviving a heart attack are much higher for people who engage in a regular aerobic exercise program.

FIGURE 7.1

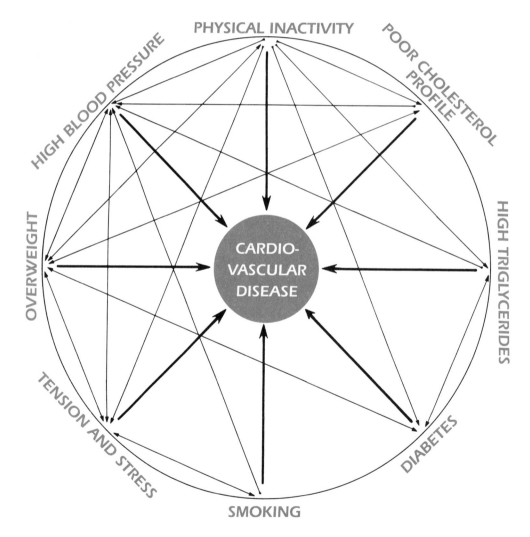

Interrelationships Among Leading Cardiovascular Risk Factors

■ *What amount of aerobic exercise is optimal for significantly decreasing the risk for cardiovascular disease?*

The required amount of exercise to maintain cardiovascular fitness is a training session approximately every 48 hours for 20 to 30 minutes in the appropriate target training zone. Although aerobic exercise definitely reduces the risk for cardiovascular problems, the amount of exercise required to offset the risk cannot be specifically pinpointed because of the many individual differences (genetic and lifestyle) between people.

According to some data, about 300 calories should be expended daily through aerobic exercise to obtain a certain degree of protection against cardiovascular disease. Dr. Ralph Paffenbarger and co-researchers' study on Harvard alumni (see Figure 1.5 in Chapter 1) found that expending 2,000 calories per week as a result of physical activity yielded the lowest risk for cardiovascular disease in this group of almost 17,000 alumni (2,000 calories per week represents about 300 calories per daily exercise session).

The work alluded to in Chapter 6 (see Figure 6.4) by Dr. Steven Blair co-workers indicated that even moderate fitness levels can substantially reduce the incidence of cardiovascular problems. The minimum dose for moderate fitness recommended under Program II in Figure 6.5 is an expenditure of about 200 calories five to seven times per week. Slightly greater protection is achieved at higher fitness levels. As noted in the previous question, nonetheless, exercise by itself is does not provide an absolute risk-free guarantee against cardiovascular disease.

■ *At what age should I start concerning myself with cardiovascular disease?*

The disease process, not only for cardiovascular disease but also cancer, starts early in life as a result of poor lifestyle habits. Studies have shown beginning stages of atherosclerosis and elevated blood lipids in children as young as 10 years old.

Many positive habits can be established early in life within the walls of your own home. If children are taught at a young age that they should avoid excessive calories, sweets, salt, tobacco, alcohol, and participate in physical activity (see Figure 7.2), their chances of leading a healthier life are much greater than is true with the present generation. Some of the best advice to humanity when it comes to teaching is: "Come and follow me." If you cultivate positive health habits in your own life, your children will be more likely to follow.

FIGURE 7.2

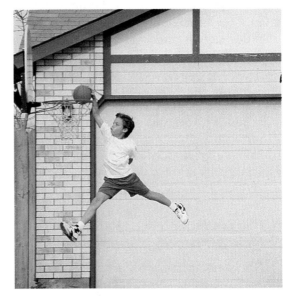

Regular physical activity during youth enhances the likelihood of lifetime participation in an exercise program.

■ *Can I exercise after donating blood?*

The average amount of blood taken in donations is about 500 ml (half liter) out of a total body volume of 5 liters. This volume is replenished immediately by reserve blood components stored in the body. Unless you are given special instructions not to exercise, there is no reason you cannot continue with your regular program.

■ *Will exercise offset the detrimental effects of cigarette smoking?*

Physical exercise often motivates toward smoking cessation but does not offset any ill effects of smoking. If anything, smoking greatly decreases the ability of the blood to transport oxygen to working muscles. Oxygen is carried in the circulatory system by hemoglobin, the iron-containing pigment of the red blood cells. Carbon monoxide, a byproduct of cigarette smoke, has 210 to 250 times greater affinity for hemoglobin than oxygen. Consequently, carbon monoxide combines much faster with hemoglobin, decreasing the oxygen-carrying capacity of the blood.

Chronic smoking also increases airway resistance, requiring the respiratory muscles to work much harder and consume more oxygen to ventilate a given amount of air. If you quit smoking, exercise does help increase the functional capacity of the pulmonary system.

■ *How can I tell if I'm exceeding the safe limits for exercise participation?*

The best method to determine whether you are exercising too strenuously is to check your heart rate and make sure it does not exceed the limits of your target zone. Exercising above this target zone may not be safe for unconditioned or high-risk individuals. You do not need to exercise beyond your target zone to gain the desired benefits for the cardiovascular system.

In addition, several physical signs will tell you when you are exceeding functional limitations. A rapid or irregular heart rate, difficult breathing, nausea, vomiting, light-headedness, headaches, dizziness, pale skin, flushness, extreme weakness, lack of energy, shakiness, sore muscles, cramps, and tightness in the chest are all signs of exercise intolerance. Learn to listen to your body. If you notice any of these symptoms, seek medical attention before continuing your exercise program.

■ *How fast should heart rate decrease following aerobic exercise?*

To a certain extent, recovery heart rate is related to fitness level. The better your cardiovascular fitness level, the faster your heart rate will decrease following exercise. As a rule of thumb, heart rate should be below 120 beats per minute 5 minutes into recovery. If your heart rate is above 120, you most likely have overexerted yourself or possibly could have some other cardiac abnormality. If you decrease the intensity or duration of exercise, or both, and you still have a fast heart rate 5 minutes into recovery, consult your physician.

■ *Do people really get a "physical high" during aerobic exercise?*

During vigorous exercise, the pituitary gland in the brain releases morphine-like substances called *endorphines*. These act not only as a pain killer but also can create feelings of euphoria and natural well-being.

Higher levels of endorphines commonly accrue from aerobic endurance activities and may remain elevated as long as 30 to 60 minutes after exercising. Many experts believe these higher levels explain the "physical high" people get during and after prolonged exercise.

How fast does a person lose the benefits of exercise after stopping an exercise program?

The time to regain the benefits of exercise differs among the various components of physical fitness and also depends on the condition the person achieves before discontinuing the exercise. Specifically with regard to cardiovascular endurance, it has been estimated that 4 weeks of aerobic training are completely reversed in 2 consecutive weeks of physical inactivity.

On the other hand, if you have been exercising regularly for months or years, 2 weeks of inactivity will not hurt you as much as it will someone who has exercised only a few weeks. As a rule of thumb, after only 48 hours of aerobic inactivity, the cardiovascular system starts to lose some of its capacity (flexibility can be maintained with two or three stretching sessions per week, and strength is easily maintained with just one maximal training session per week).

To preserve fitness, a regular exercise program, even during vacations is recommended. If you have to interrupt the program for reasons beyond your control, do not attempt to resume your training at the same level you left off but, instead, build up gradually again.

What type of clothing should I wear when I exercise?

The type of clothing you wear during exercise is important. Clothing should fit comfortably and allow free movement of the various body parts. You also should select your clothes according to air temperature and humidity. Avoid nylon and rubberized materials and tight clothes that interfere with the cooling mechanism of the human body or obstruct normal blood flow. Proper-fitting shoes, manufactured specifically for your choice of activity, also are recommended to prevent lower-limb injuries (see Figure 7.3).

FIGURE 7.3

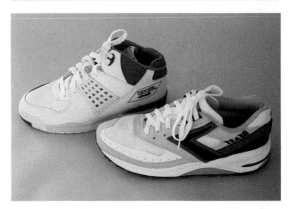

Activity-specific shoes are recommended to prevent lower extremity injuries.

What time of the day is best for exercise?

A person can exercise at almost any time of the day except about two hours following a regular meal, or the noon and early afternoon hours on hot and humid days. Many people enjoy exercising early in the morning because it gives them a good boost to start the day. Others prefer the lunch hour for weight control reasons. By exercising at noon, they do not eat as big a lunch, which helps keep daily caloric intake down. Highly stressed people seem to like the evening hours because of the relaxing effects of exercise.

■ *How long should a person wait after a meal before engaging in strenuous physical exercise?*

The length of time to wait before exercising after a meal depends on the amount of food eaten. On the average, after a regular meal a person should wait about two hours before participating in strenuous physical activity. Light physical activity, such as a walk, is fine. If anything, it helps burn extra calories and may help the body metabolize fats more efficiently.

■ *How should acute sports injuries be treated?*

The best treatment always has been prevention itself. If an activity is causing unusual discomfort or chronic irritation, attend to the cause by decreasing the intensity, switching activities, or using better equipment such as proper-fitting shoes.

In the case of an acute injury, the standard method of treatment is cold application, compression or splinting, or both, and elevation of the affected body part. Cold should be applied three to five times a day for 15 to 20 minutes at a time during the first 24 to 36 hours. This can be done by submerging the injured area in cold water or using an ice bag or applying ice massage to the affected part. Compression can be applied with an elastic bandage or wrap. Elevating the body part, whenever possible, decreases blood flow to it. The purpose of these three types of treatment is to minimize swelling in the area, which greatly increases recovery time.

After the first 36 to 48 hours, heat can be applied if no further swelling or inflammation occurs. If you have doubts regarding the nature or seriousness of the injury (such as suspected fracture), you should seek a medical evaluation.

Whenever a deformity (such as in fractures, dislocations, or partial dislocations) is obvious, splinting, cold application with an ice bag, and medical attention are required. Never try to reset any of these conditions by yourself, as you could further damage muscles, ligaments, and nerves. Treatment of these injuries always should be left to specialized medical personnel. A quick reference guide for the signs or symptoms and treatment of exercise-related problems is provided in Table 7.1.

■ *What causes muscle soreness and stiffness?*

Muscle soreness and stiffness is common in individuals who (a) begin an exercise program or participate after a long layoff from exercise, (b) exercise beyond their customary intensity and duration, and (c) perform eccentric training. The acute soreness that sets in the first few hours after exercise is thought to be related to a lack of blood (oxygen) flow and general fatigue of the exercised muscles. The delayed soreness that appears several hours after exercise (usually 12 hours or so later) and lasts 2 to 4 days may be related to actual tiny tears in muscle tissue, muscle spasms that increase fluid retention stimulating the pain nerve endings, and overstretching or tearing of connective tissue in and around muscles and joints.

Two types of contraction accompany muscular activity with movement (isotonic contractions, see Chapter 3): concentric and eccentric. During a concentric contraction the muscle shortens as it develops tension. Eccentric training involves muscular contraction with lengthening of the muscle fibers while developing tension.

For example, during the arm-curl exercise, a concentric contraction occurs when the elbow flexor muscles (biceps, brachioradialis, and brachialis) shorten as the weight is brought toward the shoulder. On the way

TABLE 7.1

Reference guide for exercise-related problems

Injury	Signs/Symptoms	Treatment*
Bruise (contusion)	Pain, swelling, discoloration	Cold application, compression, rest
Dislocations Fractures	Pain, swelling, deformity	Splinting, cold application, seek medical attention
Heat cramps	Cramps, spasms and muscle twitching in the legs, arms, and abdomen	Stop activity, get out of the heat, stretch, massage the painful area, drink plenty of fluids
Heat exhaustion	Fainting, profuse sweating, cold/clammy skin, weak/rapid pulse, weakness, headache	Stop activity, rest in a cool place, loosen clothing, rub body with cool/wet towel, drink plenty of fluids, stay out of heat for 2–3 days
Heat stroke	Hot/dry skin, no sweating, serious disorientation, rapid/full pulse, vomiting, diarrhea, unconsciousness, high body temperature	Seek immediate medical attention, request help and get out of the sun, bathe in cold water/spray with cold water/rub body with cold towels, drink plenty of cold fluids
Joint sprains	Pain, tenderness, swelling, loss of use, discoloration	Cold application, compression, elevation, rest, heat after 36 to 48 hours (if no further swelling)
Muscle cramps	Pain, spasm	Stretch muscle(s), use mild exercises for involved area
Muscle soreness and stiffness	Tenderness, pain	Mild stretching, low-intensity exercise, warm bath
Muscle strains	Pain, tenderness, swelling, loss of use	Cold application, compression, elevation, rest, heat after 36 to 48 hours (if no further swelling)
Shin splints	Pain, tenderness	Cold application prior to and following any physical activity, rest, heat (if no activity is carried out)
Side stitch	Pain on the side of the abdomen below the rib cage	Decrease level of physical activity or stop altogether, gradually increase level of fitness
Tendonitis	Pain, tenderness, loss of use	Rest, cold application, heat after 48 hours

* Cold should be applied 3 to 4 times a day for 15 minutes
   Heat can be applied 3 times a day for 15 to 20 minutes

down, the muscles contract eccentrically as they lengthen while the person slowly lowers the weight to the starting position. Similarly, running downhill requires eccentric contractions in the leg muscles and level running requires concentric contractions. Eccentric training has been shown to produce greater muscle soreness than concentric training.

To prevent soreness and stiffness, the recommended approach is to stretch adequately before and after exercise and to progress gradually into your exercise program. Do not attempt to do too much too quickly. If you become sore and stiff, mild stretching, low-intensity exercise to stimulate blood flow, and a warm bath can help relieve the pain.

Stretching may be of greatest significance following exercise. Tired muscles tend to contract to a shorter than normal length. By-products of exercise metabolism also may cause muscle spasms. Post-exercise stretching thus can help return a muscle to its normal length.

■ *How should I care for shin splints?*

One of the most common injuries to the lower limbs is the shin splint. It is characterized by pain and irritation in the shin region of the leg and usually results from one or more of the following: (a) lack of proper and gradual conditioning, (b) doing physical activities on hard surfaces (wooden floors, hard tracks, cement, and asphalt), (c) fallen arches in the feet, (d) chronic overuse, (e) muscle fatigue, (f) faulty posture, (g) improper shoes, and (h) excessively overweight while participating in weight-bearing activities.

Shin splints may be managed by: (a) removing or reducing the cause (exercising on softer surfaces, wearing better shoes or arch supports, or completely stopping exercise until

the shin splints heal); (b) doing mild stretching exercises before and after physical activity; (c) using ice massage for 10 to 20 minutes before and after physical participation; and (d) applying active heat (whirlpool and hot baths) for 15 minutes, two to three times a day. In addition, supportive taping during physical activity is helpful (a qualified athletic trainer can readily teach you the proper taping technique).

■ *What causes side stitch?*

Side stitch happens primarily in the early stages of exercise participation. The exact cause of this sharp pain that sometimes occurs during exercise is unknown. Some experts suggest that it could relate to a lack of blood flow to the respiratory muscles during strenuous physical exertion. This stitch seems to occur only in unconditioned beginners or trained individuals when they exercise at higher intensities than usual. As the physical condition improves, this problem disappears unless training is intensified. If this is a problem for you, slow down, and if it persists, stop altogether.

■ *What causes muscle cramps, and what should be done when they occur?*

Muscle cramps are caused by the body's depletion of essential electrolytes or a breakdown in the coordination between opposing muscle groups. If you have a muscle cramp, first attempt to stretch the muscles involved. In the case of the calf muscle, for example, pull your toes up toward the knees. After stretching the muscles, gently rub them down, and finally do some mild exercises requiring the use of those particular muscles.

In pregnant and lactating women, muscle cramps often are related to a lack of calcium. If women get cramps during these times, calcium supplements usually relieve the problem. Tight clothing also can cause cramps because it restricts blood flow to active muscle tissue.

■ *Why is exercising in hot and humid conditions unsafe?*

When a person exercises, only 30–40% of the energy the body produces is used for mechanical work or movement. The rest of the energy (60–70%) is converted into heat. If this heat cannot be dissipated properly because the weather is too hot or the relative humidity is too high, body temperature increases, and in extreme cases can result in death.

The specific heat of body tissue (the heat required to raise the temperature of the body by one degree Centigrade) is .38 calories per pound of body weight per one degree Centigrade (.38 cal/lb/°C). This indicates that if no body heat is dissipated, a 150-pound person has to burn only 58.5 calories (150 × .38) to increase total body temperature by one degree Centigrade. If this person were to engage in an exercise session requiring 300 calories (about 3 miles running) without dissipating any heat, the inner body temperature would increase by 5.3 degrees Centigrade, the equivalent of going from 98.6 to 108.1 degrees Fahrenheit (°F)!

This example clearly illustrates the need for caution when exercising in hot or humid weather. If the relative humidity is too high, body heat cannot be lost through evaporation because the atmosphere already is saturated with water vapor. In one instance, a football casualty occurred at a temperature of only 64 degrees Fahrenheit but at a relative humidity of 100%. As a general rule, care must be taken when air temperature is above 90 degrees and the relative humidity is above 60%.

The American College of Sports Medicine has recommended that individuals should not engage in strenuous physical activity when the readings of a wet bulb globe thermometer exceed 82.4 degrees Fahrenheit. With this type of thermometer, the wet bulb is cooled by evaporation, and on dry days it shows a lower temperature than the regular (dry) thermometer. On humid days the cooling effect is less because of decreased evaporation; hence, the difference between the wet and dry readings is not as great.

The American Running and Fitness Association offers the following descriptions and first-aid measures for the three major signs of trouble when exercising in the heat:

Heat cramps symptoms include cramps, spasms and muscle twitching in the legs, arms, and abdomen. To relieve heat cramps, stop exercising, get out of the heat, massage the painful area, slowly stretch, and drink plenty of fluids.

Heat exhaustion symptoms include fainting; dizziness; profuse sweating; cold, clammy skin; weakness; headache; and a rapid, weak pulse. If you incur any of these symptoms, stop and find a cool place to rest. Drink plenty of cool fluids. Loosen or remove clothing, and rub your body with a cool, wet towel. Stay out of the heat for the rest of the day, and possibly for the next two or three days.

Heat stroke symptoms include serious disorientation; warm, dry skin; no sweating; rapid, full pulse; vomiting; diarrhea; unconsciousness; and high body temperature. As the body temperature climbs, unexplained anxiety sets in. When the body temperature reaches 104 to 105 degrees Fahrenheit, the individual may feel a cold sensation in the trunk of the body, goose bumps, nausea, throbbing in the temples, and numbness in the extremities. Most people become incoherent after this stage. When body temperature reaches 105 to 106 degrees, disorientation, loss of fine-motor control, and muscular weakness set in. If the temperature exceeds 106 degrees, serious neurologic injury and death may be imminent.

Heat stroke requires immediate emergency medical attention. Request help and get out of the sun. While you're waiting to be taken to the hospital's emergency room, your body should be sprayed with cool water and rubbed with cool towels. You also should be fanned and given plenty of cold liquids.

■ *What are the recommended guidelines for fluid replacement during prolonged aerobic exercise?*

The main objective of fluid replacement during prolonged aerobic exercise is to maintain the blood volume so circulation and sweating can continue at normal levels. Adequate water replacement is the most important factor in preventing heat disorders. Drinking about 8 ounces of cool water every 10 to 15 minutes during exercise seems ideal to prevent dehydration. Cold fluids seem to be absorbed more rapidly from the stomach.

Commercial fluid replacement solutions (e.g., Take-Five, Gatorade) contain about 5% glucose, which slows down water absorption during exercise in the heat. During prolonged aerobic exercise in cool environments, commercially prepared solutions may be helpful because not as much water is lost through the sweating mechanism. After drinking a glucose solution, the sugar does not become available to the muscles for about 30 minutes. Drinking solutions with a sugar concentration higher than 5% significantly slows down water absorption from the stomach.

■ *What precautions must be taken when exercising in the cold?*

As contrasted with hot and humid conditions, exercising in the cold usually is not health-threatening because clothing for heat conservation can be selected and exercise itself increases body heat production. The popular belief that exercising in cold temperatures (32 degrees Fahrenheit and lower) freezes the lungs is false because the air is warmed properly in the air passages before it ever reaches the lungs. Cold is not what poses a threat but, rather, wind velocity, which greatly affects the chill factor. For example, exercising at a temperature of 25 degrees Fahrenheit with adequate clothing is not too cold, but if the wind is blowing at 25 miles per hour, the chill factor reduces the actual temperature to minus five degrees Fahrenheit. This effect is even worse if the person is wet and exhausted.

When exercising in the cold, you have to protect the face, head, hands, and feet, as they may be subject to frostbite even when the lungs are under no risk. In cold temperatures, about 30% of the body's heat is lost through the head's surface area, if unprotected. Wearing several layers of lightweight clothing is preferable to one single, thick layer, because warm air is trapped between layers of clothes, conserving more heat.

SPECIAL CONSIDERATIONS FOR WOMEN

■ *Physiological differences between men and women*

Men and women have several basic differences that affect physical performance. On the average, men are about 3 to 4 inches taller and 25 to 30 pounds heavier. The average body fat in college males is about 12 to 16%, whereas in college females it is 22 to 26%.

Maximal oxygen uptake (aerobic capacity) is about 15 to 30% greater in men, primarily related to a higher hemoglobin concentration and a lower body fat content in men. The higher hemoglobin concentration allows men to carry a greater amount of oxygen during exercise, which is advantageous during aerobic events.

The quality of muscle in men and women is the same. Men, however, are stronger because they have a greater amount of muscle mass and a greater capacity for muscle hypertrophy (the muscle's ability to increase in size). The larger capacity for muscle hypertrophy is related to sex-specific hormones. Strength differences, nevertheless, are significantly less when taking into consideration body size and composition.

Men also have wider shoulders, longer extremities, and a 10% greater bone width, except for pelvic width. Although there are gender differences in physiological characteristics, both respond to training in a similar way.

■ *If the potential for muscle hypertrophy in women is not as great, why do so many women body builders develop such heavy musculature?*

Masculinity and femininity are established by genetic inheritance and not by the amount of physical activity. Variations in the extent of masculinity and femininity are determined by individual differences in hormonal secretions of androgen, testosterone, estrogen, and progesterone. Women with a bigger-than-average build are inclined to participate in sports because of their natural physical advantage. As a result, many women have associated sports and strength participation with large muscle size.

In the sport of body building, athletes follow intense training routines consisting of two or more hours of constant weight lifting with short rest intervals between sets. Many times during the training routine, they perform back-to-back exercises using the same muscle groups. The objective of this type of training is to "pump" extra blood into the muscles, which makes the muscles appear much bigger than they really are in resting conditions. Based on intensity and length of the training session, the muscles can remain filled with blood, appearing measurably larger for several hours after completing the training session. In real life, these women are not as muscular as they seem when they are "pumped up" for a contest.

A big point of controversy in body building is the use of anabolic steroids and human growth hormones, even among women participants. Anabolic steroids are synthetic versions of the male sex hormone testosterone, which promotes muscle development and hypertrophy. These hormones, however, produce detrimental and undesirable side effects (such as hypertension, fluid retention, decreased breast size, deepening voice, facial whiskers, and body hair growth), which some women deem tolerable. According to several sports medicine physicians and women body builders, about 80% of female body builders have used steroids. Some women's track-and-field coaches have indicated that as many as 95% of women athletes in this sport around the world used anabolic steroids to remain competitive at the international level.

Women who take steroids certainly will build heavy musculature, and if they take steroids long enough, it will produce masculinizing effects. As a result, the International Federation of Body Building instituted a mandatory steroid-testing program among women participating in the Miss Olympia contest. When drugs are not used to promote development, improved body image is the rule rather than the exception in women who participate in body building, strength training, and sports in general (see Figure 7.4).

FIGURE 7.4

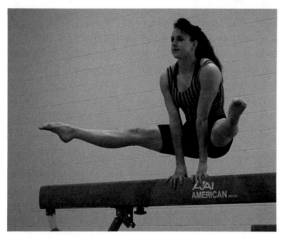

Contrary to some beliefs, high levels of strength do not lead to large muscle size in women.

■ *Does exercise participation hinder menstruation?*

In some instances highly trained athletes may develop amenorrhea (cessation of menstruation) during training and competition. This condition is seen frequently in extremely lean women who also engage in sports requiring strenuous physical effort over a sustained period of time, but it is by no means irreversible. Whether the condition is caused by physical or emotional stress related to high-intensity training, excessively low body fat, or other factors is unknown at this time

Although, on the average, women have less physical capacity during menstruation, they have broken Olympic and world records at all stages of the menstrual cycle, according to medical surveys taken at the Olympic games. Menstruation should not keep a woman from participating in athletics, and it does not necessarily have a negative impact on performance.

■ *Does exercise help relieve dysmenorrhea (painful menstruation)?*

Exercise has not been shown to either cure or aggravate painful menstruation, but it has been shown to relieve menstrual cramps because of improved circulation to the uterus. Less severe menstrual cramps also could be related to higher levels of endorphines produced during prolonged physical activity, which may counteract pain.

■ *Is exercising during pregnancy safe?*

Women should not hesitate to exercise during pregnancy. If anything, they should exercise to strengthen the body and prepare for delivery. Some reports indicate that physically fit women appear to have shorter labor, easier delivery, and faster recovery than unfit women do.

Pregnant women in American Indian tribes continue to carry out all of their difficult work chores up to the very day of delivery, and a few hours after giving birth, they resume their normal activities. Several women athletes have competed in various sports during the early stages of pregnancy. At the 1952 Olympic games, a pregnant woman won a bronze medal in track and field. In any event, the woman and her personal physician should make the final decision regarding her exercise program.

Experts recommend that women who have exercised regularly may continue to carry out the same activity through the fifth month of pregnancy. They should take care, however, not to exceed a body (core) temperature of 38.5 degrees Centigrade (101.3 degrees Fahrenheit). To ensure adequate oxygen delivery to the baby, exercise heart rates should be kept below 140 beats per minute, and training sessions should be limited to 15 minutes. After the fifth month, walking, stationary cycling, and moderate swimming and water aerobics are suggested in conjunction with some light strengthening exercises. For women who have not exercised regularly, 20 to 30 minutes of daily walking and light strengthening exercises are recommended throughout the pregnancy.

■ *What is osteoporosis and how can it be prevented?*

Osteoporosis is the softening, deterioration, or loss of total body bone. Bones become so weak and brittle that the person is vulnerable to fractures, primarily of the hip, wrist, and spine. Osteoporosis is really a preventable condition. The process slowly begins in the third and fourth decade of life.

The importance of normal estrogen levels, adequate calcium intake, and physical activity cannot be overemphasized in maximizing bone density in young women and lowering the rate of bone loss later in life. All three factors are crucial in preventing osteoporosis. The absence of any one of these three factors leads to bone loss, for which the other two never completely compensate.

Prevention of osteoporosis begins early in life by having enough calcium in the diet (RDA of 800 to 1,200 mg per day) and by participating in a lifetime exercise program. Also, vitamin D, which is necessary for optimal calcium absorption, may have to be supplemented. A list of selected foods and their respective calcium content is provided in Table 7.2.

TABLE 7.2

Lowfat calcium-rich foods

Food	Amount	Calcium (mg)	Calories	Calories from Fat
Beans, red kidney, cooked	1 cup	70	218	4%
Beet, greens, cooked	1/2 cup	72	13	—
Broccoli, cooked, drained	1 sm stalk	123	36	—
Burrito, bean	1	173	307	28%
Cottage cheese, 2% lowfat	1/2 cup	78	103	18%
Milk, nonfat, powdered	1 tbsp	52	27	1%
Milk, skim	1 cup	296	88	3%
Ice milk (vanilla)	1/2 cup	102	100	27%
Instant breakfast, whole milk	1 cup	301	280	26%
Kale, cooked, drained	1/2 cup	103	22	—
Okra, cooked, drained	1/2 cup	74	23	—
Shrimp, boiled	3 oz.	99	99	9%
Spinach, raw	1 cup	51	14	—
Yogurt, fruit	1 cup	345	231	8%
Yogurt, lowfat, plain	1 cup	271	160	20%

Weight-bearing exercise such as walking, jogging, and weight training are especially helpful. Not only do they tone up muscles, but they also produce stronger and thicker bones.

Prevailing research tells us that estrogen is the most important factor in preventing bone loss. Lumbar bone density in women with regular menstrual cycles exceeds that of women with a history of oligomenorrhea (irregular cycles) and amenorrhea (cessation of menstruation) interspaced with regular cycles. Furthermore, the lumbar density of these two groups of women is higher than that of women who never had regular cycles.

Women are especially susceptible to osteoporosis after menopause because of accompanying estrogen loss, hastens the rate at which bone mass is broken down. Following menopause, every woman should consider hormone replacement therapy and discuss it with her physician. Women who have estrogen therapy do not lose bone mineral density at the rate non-therapy women do. Neither exercise nor calcium supplementation will offset the damaging effects of lower estrogen levels.

■ *Do women have special iron needs?*

Iron is a key element of hemoglobin in blood, which carries oxygen from the lungs to all bodily tissues. The RDA of iron for adult women is 15 mg per day (10 mg for men). A survey by the U. S. Department of Agriculture revealed that 19- to 50-year-old women in the United States, unfortunately, consumed only 60% of the U.S. RDA for iron. People who do not have enough iron in the body can develop iron deficiency anemia, in which the concentration of hemoglobin in the red blood cells is less than it should be.

Physically active women also may have a greater than average iron need. Heavy training is thought to create an iron demand higher than the recommended intake because

small amounts of iron are lost through sweat, urine, and stools. Mechanical trauma, caused by pounding the feet on pavement during extensive jogging, may also lead to the destruction of iron-containing red blood cells. A large percentage of female endurance athletes have iron deficiency. Blood ferritin levels, a measure of stored iron in the human body, should be checked frequently in women who participate in intense physical training.

Rates of iron absorption and iron loss vary from person to person. In most cases, though, people can get enough iron by eating more iron-rich foods such as beans, peas, green leafy vegetables, enriched grain products, egg yolk, fish, and lean meats (organ meats are especially good sources, but they also are high in cholesterol). A list of foods high in iron content is given in Table 7.3.

NUTRITION AND WEIGHT CONTROL QUESTIONS

■ *What is the difference between a calorie and a kilocalorie (kcal)?*

Calorie is the unit of measure indicating the energy value of food and cost of physical activity. Technically, a kilocalorie (kcal) or large calorie is the amount of heat necessary to raise the temperature of one kilogram of water one degree Centigrade, but for simplification, people call it a calorie rather than kcal. For example, if the caloric value of a food is 100 calories (kcal), the energy in this food could raise the temperature of 100 kilograms of water by 1 degree Centigrade.

■ *Does cooking affect the amount of calories in food?*

Cooking does not significantly alter the caloric content of food. The only exception is

TABLE 7.3

Iron-rich foods

Food	Amount	Iron (mg)	Calories	Choles-terol	Calories from Fat
Beans, red kidney, cooked	1 cup	4.4	218	0	4%
Beef, ground lean	3 oz.	3.0	186	81	48%
Beef, sirloin	3 oz.	2.5	329	77	74%
Beef, liver, fried	3 oz.	7.5	195	345	42%
Beet, greens, cooked	1/2 cup	1.4	13	0	—
Broccoli, cooked, drained	1 sm stalk	1.1	36	0	—
Burrito, bean	1	2.4	307	14	28%
Egg, hard, cooked	1	1.0	72	250	63%
Farina (Cream of Wheat), cooked	1/2 cup	6.0	51	0	—
Instant breakfast, whole milk	1 cup	8.0	280	33	26%
Peas, frozen, cooked, drained	1/2 cup	1.5	55	0	—
Shrimp, boiled	3 oz.	2.7	99	128	9%
Spinach, raw	1 cup	1.7	14	0	—
Vegetables, mixed, cooked	1 cup	2.4	116	0	—

meat, in which broiling and barbecuing drain off some of the fat and decrease the caloric content. Frying, on the other hand, significantly increases the caloric content of food because of the large number of calories in the oil in which the food is fried.

■ *Why do some people gain weight rather than lose weight after they begin an exercise program?*

Physical exercise leads to an increase in lean body mass. Therefore, body weight often remains the same or increases after starting an exercise program. At the same time, inches and percent body fat decrease. The increase in lean tissue results in an increased functional capacity. With exercise, most of the weight (fat) loss is seen after a few weeks of training, when the lean component has stabilized.

"Skinny" people should realize that the only healthy way to increase body weight is through exercise, primarily strength-training exercises. Attempting to gain weight by just eating more will increase the fat component and not the lean component, which is not conducive to better health. Consequently, exercise is the best solution to weight (fat) reduction as well as weight (lean) gain.

■ *Are rubberized sweatsuits and steam baths effective in losing weight?*

The answer to this question is simply no! When a person wears a sweatsuit or steps into a sauna, the resulting weight lost is not fat but merely a significant amount of water. Sure, it looks nice when you step on the scale immediately afterward, but this represents a false loss of weight. As soon as you replace body fluids, you quickly gain back the weight. Wearing rubberized sweatsuits not only hastens the rate of vital body fluid loss, but at the same time it raises core temperature. This combination puts a person in danger of dehydration, which impairs cellular function and in extreme cases can even cause death.

■ *Can cellulite be decreased with special exercises?*

There is no such thing as spot reducing or losing "cellulite," as some people refer to the fat deposits that bulge out on certain body parts. These deposits are nothing more than enlarged fat cells from accumulated body fat. Just doing several sets of daily sit-ups will not get rid of fat in the midsection of the body. Fat comes off throughout the entire body, not just the exercised area. The greatest proportion of fat may come off the biggest fat deposits, but the caloric output of a few sets of sit-ups has no real effect on reducing total body fat. A person has to exercise much longer to actually see results.

The only effective way to decrease body fat is through a combined lifetime food selection program and a regular exercise program. You will need willpower, patience, and persistence. If you really try, it will work. The best tip is to keep the weight (fat) off rather than let it go and try to control it once it has crept up on you. Only one person in 200 is able to keep the weight off after a successful weight-loss

program. The few who succeed are those who implement lifetime changes in food selection and physical activity. As more people become educated and apply these two basic principles, the rate of success will improve.

■ *Are mechanical vibrators useful in losing weight?*

Some people will try almost anything to lose weight as long as they can still overindulge. These people can be easily deceived and often resort to quick fixes in an attempt to solve their weight problem. Mechanical vibrators are worthless in a weight control program. Vibrating belts and turning rollers may feel good, but they require no effort whatsoever. According to one report, a person would have to continuously vibrate for 76 hours to lose the equivalent of one pound of fat! Fat cannot be "shaken off"; it is used by the body as an energy substrate and it is lost most efficiently by burning it in muscle tissue.

■ *How detrimental are coffee and alcohol to good health?*

Caffeine and alcohol are drugs, and as such can produce several undesirable side effects. Caffeine doses of more than 200 to 500 mg can cause an inordinately rapid heart rate, abnormal heart rhythms, a rise in blood pressure, higher body temperature, and oversecretion of gastric acids, leading to stomach problems. It also may have some link to birth defects in unborn children. It, too, may induce symptoms of anxiety, depression, nervousness, and dizziness. The caffeine content of various types of coffee ranges from 65 mg per 6 ounces for instant coffee to as high as 180 mg for drip coffee. Soft drinks, mainly colas, range in caffeine content from 30 to 60 mg per 12-ounce can.

Alcohol intake cuts down on peripheral vision, impairs the ability to see and hear, causes slower reactions, reduces concentration and motor performance (including swaying and poor judgment of distance and speed of moving objects), decreases fear, increases risk-taking behaviors, causes more frequent urination, and induces sleep. A single large dose of alcohol may also lower sexual function.

One of the most unpleasant, dangerous, and life-threatening consequences of drinking is the synergistic action of alcohol when combined with other drugs, particularly central nervous system depressants. The effects of mixing alcohol with another drug can be much greater than the sum of two drug actions by themselves. Individuals react to a combination of alcohol and other drugs in different ways, ranging from loss of consciousness to death.

Long-term manifestations of alcohol abuse can be serious and life-threatening. Some of the harmful effects are cirrhosis of the liver (scarring of the liver, often fatal); greater risk for oral, esophageal, and liver cancer; cardiomyopathy (a disease that affects the heart muscle); high blood pressure; greater risk for strokes; inflammation of the esophagus, stomach, small intestine, and pancreas; stomach ulcers; sexual impotence; malnutrition; brain cell damage and consequent loss of memory; psychosis; depression; and hallucinations.

The negative effects of long-term caffeine and alcohol consumption, even in moderate amounts, are more detrimental to health and well-being than any short-term pleasures derived from their consumption.

■ Do athletes or individuals who train for long periods need a special diet?

Many people have thought that highly trained individuals need a special diet to be successful in their sport. The simple truth is that unless the diet is deficient in basic nutrients, no special, secret, or magic diets will help a person perform better or develop faster as a result of what he or she eats. As long as the diet is balanced (is based on a large variety of foods from each of the basic food groups), athletes do not need any supplements. Even in strength training and body building no additional protein in excess of 20% of total daily caloric intake is necessary.

The only difference between a sedentary person and a highly trained one is in the total number of calories required daily. The trained person may take in more calories because he or she expends more energy in intense physical training.

The only time a normal diet should be modified is when someone is going to participate in long-distance events of more than an hour (for example, marathon, triathlon, road cycling). Athletic performance is enhanced for these types of events through a regular balanced diet along with intensive physical training during the fifth and fourth days before the event, followed by a diet high in carbohydrates (about 70%) and a gradual decrease in training intensity the three days before the event.

EXERCISE AND AGING

■ Exercise programs for older adults

Unlike any time before in American society, the elderly population constitutes the fastest growing segment in the United States. In 1880, less than 3% of the total population — fewer than 2 million people — were older than 65. By 1980, the elderly population had reached about 25 million, representing more than 11.3% of the population. It has been estimated that the elderly will make up more than 20% of the total population by the year 2035.

Older adults have been neglected in fitness programs designed for them, even though fitness is just as important for older people as it is for the young. Older individuals who are physically fit benefit like everyone else from better health and a higher quality of life.

The main objective of fitness programs for older adults should be to improve their functional capacity. According to a committee of the American Alliance of Health, Physical Education, Recreation, and Dance (AAHPERD), functional fitness for older adults means the individual's physical capacity to meet ordinary and unexpected demands of daily life safely and effectively.

This definition points out the need for fitness programs that closely relate to typical activities of this population. The AAHPERD committee encourages programs that will help develop cardiovascular endurance, localized muscular endurance, muscular flexibility, agility and balance, and motor coordination. A battery of fitness tests for older adults can be obtained from the AAHPERD national office in Reston, Virginia.

■ What is the relationship between aging and physical work capacity?

Lack of physical activity, a common phenomenon in our society as people age, may cause lower physical work capacity that is far more influential than the effects of aging itself. Data on individuals who have been physically active throughout life suggest that these people have a higher level of functional capacity and do not succumb to typical declines in later years. Dr. George Sheehan, cardiologist and runner, states that, from a functional point of view, the typical American is 30 years older than his or her chronological age indicates. Translated into an example, an active 60-year-old person can have a work capacity similar to that of a sedentary 30-year-old individual.

Unfortunately, unhealthy behaviors precipitate premature aging. Productive life for sedentary people ends at about age 60. Most of them hope to live to age 65 or 70 and often must cope with serious physical ailments. "These people stop living at age 60 but choose to be buried at age 70." Scientists believe that a healthy lifestyle allows people to live a vibrant life — a physically, intellectually, emotionally, and socially active existence — to age 95. When death comes to active people, it usually comes rather quickly and not as a result of prolonged illness (see Figure 7.5). Such are the rewards of a wellness way of life.

■ Do older adults respond to physical training?

The trainability of elderly men and women alike and the effectiveness of physical activity have been demonstrated through research. Older adults who become more physically active gain in cardiovascular endurance, strength, and flexibility. The extent of improvement depends on their initial fitness level and the types of activities selected for their training (walking, cycling, strength training, and so on).

Improvements in maximal oxygen uptake in older adults are similar to those of younger people, although older people seem to require a longer training period to achieve these changes. Declines in endurance (maximal oxygen uptake) per decade of life after age 25 seem to be about 9% for sedentary adults and 5% or less in active people.

Results from a study on the effects of aging on the cardiovascular system of male exercisers versus non-exercisers, showed that the maximal oxygen uptake of regular exercisers is almost twice that of the non-exercisers. Between ages 50 and 68, maximal oxygen uptake declined only 13% in the active group, compared to 41% in the inactive group. These changes suggest that a third of the loss in

FIGURE 7.5

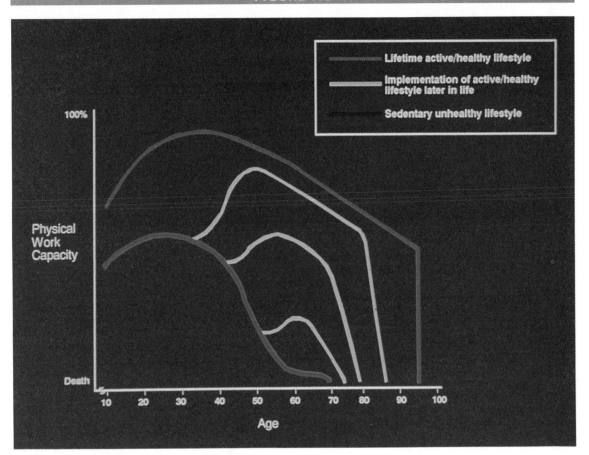

Relationship between physical work capacity, aging, and lifestyle habits.

maximal oxygen uptake is from aging and two-thirds of the loss comes from inactivity. Blood pressure, heart rate, and body weight also were remarkably better in the exercising group.

In strength development, older adults can increase their strength levels, but the amount of muscle hypertrophy achieved decreases with age. Strength gains as high as 200% have been found in previously inactive adults over the age of 90. In terms of body composition, after age 60, inactive adults continue to gain body fat despite the tendency toward lower body weight.

Older adults who wish to take part in an exercise program should have a complete medical exam, including a stress electrocardiogram test. Recommended activities for older adults include calisthenics, walking, jogging, swimming, cycling, and water aerobics. They should not do isometric and very intense weight training exercises. Activities that require all-out effort and those that require participants to hold their breath (valsalva maneuver) tend to decrease blood flow to the heart and cause blood pressure to go up, placing a bigger load on the heart. Older adults should take part in activities that require continuous and rhythmic muscular activity (about 50% to 70% of functional capacity), as these activities do not cause blood pressure to jump or cause excessive strain on the heart.

As illustrated in Figure 7.5, physical fitness or physical work capacity can be increased at any age. Complete benefits of a healthy lifestyle, nonetheless, are best attained by starting early in life.

WHAT'S NEXT NOW THAT I'VE COMPLETED THE ASSIGNMENTS IN THIS BOOK?

The objective of this book is to provide you with the information necessary to implement your personal fitness and wellness program. If you have read and successfully completed your assignments, including a regular exercise program, you should be convinced of the value of exercise and healthy lifestyle habits in achieving total well-being.

Now that you are about to finish this course, the real challenge is a lifetime commitment to fitness and wellness. Adhering to the program in a structured setting is a lot easier. Nonetheless, as you continue with your personal program, keep in mind that the greatest benefit of fitness and wellness is to improve the quality of your life. Most people who engage in a personal fitness and wellness program recognize this new quality of life after only a few weeks of training and practicing healthy lifestyle patterns. In some instances, especially individuals who led a poor lifestyle for a long time, establishing positive habits and gaining feelings of well-being might take a few months. In the end, however, everyone who applies the principles of fitness and wellness will reap the desired benefits. Being diligent and taking control of yourself will provide you a better, happier, healthier, and more productive life. And once you get there, you won't want to have it any other way.

Pre- and Post-Fitness Profiles

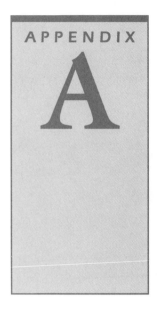

FIGURE A.1

Personal Fitness Profile: Pre-Test

Date: ______________ Course: ______________ Section: ______________

Name: ______________________________ Age: ________ Male or Female: M / F

Body Weight: ________ . ________

Fitness Component	Test Data	Test Results	Fitness Classification	Fitness Goal
Cardiovascular Endurance	Time	$VO_{2\,max.}$		$VO_{2\,max.}$
1.5-Mile Run	____ : ____	____ . ____	________	____ . ____
	Time			
1.0-Mile Walk	____ : ____			
	Heat Rate	$VO_{2\,max.}$		$VO_{2\,max.}$
	________	____ . ____	________	____ . ____
Muscular Strength / Endurance	Reps	Percentile		
Bench Jumps	________	________	________	________
Chair Dips / Mod. Push-Ups	________	________	________	________
Abdominal Curl-Ups	________	________	________	________
Average Percentile		________	________	
Muscular Flexibility	Inches	Percentile		
Modified Sit-and-Reach	________	________	________	________
Body Rotation (R/L)	________	________	________	________
Average Percentile		________	________	
Body Composition	mm			
Chest / Triceps	________			
Abdominal / Suprailium	________			
Thith	________			
Sum of Skinfolds	________			
Percent Body Fat		________	________	________
Lean Body Mass (lbs.)		________		________

FIGURE A.2

Personal Fitness Profile: Post-Test

Date: _____ Course: _____ Section: _____

Name: _____ Age: _____ Male or Female: M / F

Body Weight: _____ . _____

Fitness Component	Test Data	Test Results	Fitness Classification
Cardiovascular Endurance	Time	VO₂ max.	
1.5-Mile Run	_____ : _____	_____ . _____	_____
	Time		
1.0-Mile Walk	_____ : _____		
	Heat Rate	VO₂ max.	
	_____	_____ . _____	_____
Muscular Strength / Endurance	Reps	Percentile	
Bench Jumps	_____	_____	_____
Chair Dips / Mod. Push-Ups	_____	_____	_____
Abdominal Curl-Ups	_____	_____	_____
Average Percentile		_____	_____
Muscular Flexibility	Inches	Percentile	
Modified Sit-and-Reach	_____	_____	_____
Body Rotation (R/L)	_____	_____	_____
Average Percentile		_____	_____
Body Composition	mm		
Chest / Triceps	_____		
Abdominal / Suprailium	_____		
Thith	_____		
Sum of Skinfolds	_____		
Percent Body Fat		_____	_____
Lean Body Mass (lbs.)		_____	_____

FIGURE A.3

Computerized Fitness Profile: Pre- and Post-Test Comparison*

```
                            FITNESS PROFILE

                  Based on the textbook Fitness and Wellness
                   by Werner W.K. Hoeger and Sharon A. Hoeger
                           Morton Publishing Company
                             Englewood, Colorado


James Doe                                 Course: PE 114: Fitness Foundations
Age: 18                                   Section: 01
Gender: M                                 Instructor: Werner Hoeger
```

Test Item	Most Recent Test 09-22-1992	Current Test 12-14-1992	Current Fitness Rating	Percent Change
Cardiovascular Endurance (1.5-mile run test)	39.8 ml/kg/min	45.8 ml/kg/min	Good	+15
Muscular Endurance	37 %tile	60 %tile	Good	
Number of bench jumps	48 reps – 30 %tile	56 reps – 60 %tile	Good	+17
Number of chair dips	27 reps – 60 %tile	32 reps – 80 %tile	Excellent	+19
Number of curl-ups	17 reps – 20 %tile	26 reps – 40 %tile	Average	+53
Muscular Flexibility	50 %tile	50 %tile	Average	
Sit and reach	16.5 in – 70 %tile	17.5 in – 70 %tile	Good	+6
Right body rotation	15.5 in – 30 %tile	17.0 in – 30 %tile	Fair	+10
Body Composition				
Percent body fat	23.7 %	21.4 %	Overweight	–10
Recommended percent body fat		20.0 %		
Body weight	175.0 lbs	170.5 lbs		
Recommended body weight		167.5 lbs		

*Computer software is available from Morton Publishing Company, Englewood, Colorado.

Strength Training Exercises

Strength-Training Exercises Without Weights

Step-Up

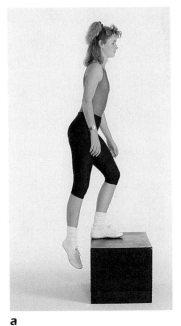

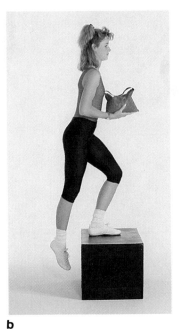

a   b

Action: Step up and down using a box or chair approximately twelve to fifteen inches high. Conduct one set using the same leg each time you go up and then conduct a second set using the other leg. You could also alternate legs on each step-up cycle. You may increase the resistance by holding a child or some other object in your arms (hold the child or object close to the body to avoid increased strain in the lower back).

Muscles Developed: Gluteal muscles, quadriceps, gastrocnemius, and soleus.

Photographs for Exercises 11, 13, 16, and 17 are courtesy of Universal Gym® Equipment, Inc., 930 27th Avenue, S.W., Cedar Rapids, IA 52406. Photographs for Exercises 12, 14, and 15 are courtesy of Nautilus®, a registered trademark of Nautilus® Sports/Medical Industries, Inc., P.O. Box 809014, Dallas, TX 75380-9014.

EXERCISE 2

High-Jumper

Action: Start with the knees bent at approximately 150° and jump as high as you can, raising both arms simultaneously.

Muscles Developed: Gluteal muscles, quadriceps, gastrocnemius, and soleus.

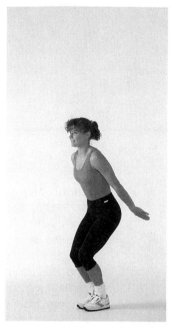
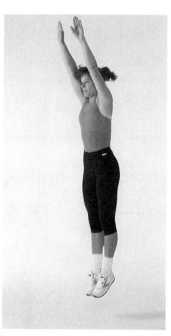

a   b

EXERCISE 3

Push-Up

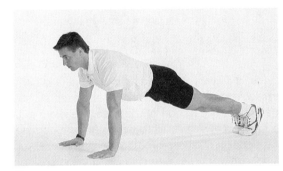

a

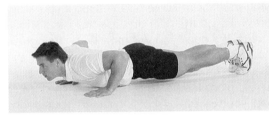

b

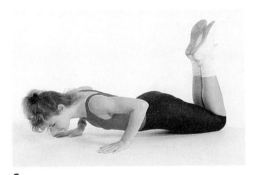

c

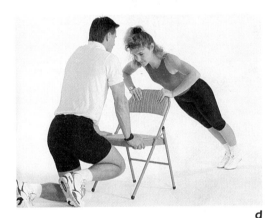

d

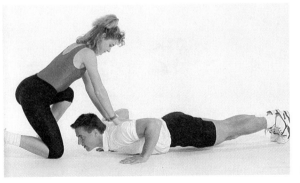

e

Action: Maintaining your body as straight as possible, flex the elbows, lowering the body until you almost touch the floor, then raise yourself back up to the starting position. If you are unable to perform the push-up as indicated, you can decrease the resistance by supporting the lower body with the knees rather than the feet (see illustration c) or using an incline plane and supporting your hands at a higher point than the floor (see illustration d). If you wish to increase the resistance, have someone else add resistance to your shoulders as you are coming back up (see illustration e).

Muscles Developed: Triceps, deltoid, pectoralis major, erector spinae, and abdominals.

EXERCISE 4

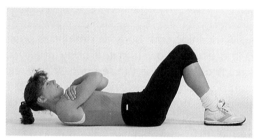

a

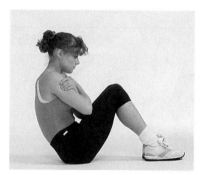

b

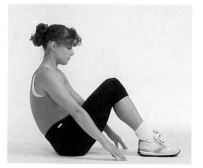

c

Abdominal Crunch and Abdominal Curl-Up

Action: Start with your head and shoulders off the floor, arms crossed on your chest, and knees slightly bent (the greater the flexion of the knee, the more difficult the sit-up). Now curl up to about 30° (abdominal crunch — see illustration b) or curl all the way up (abdominal curl-up), then return to the starting position without letting the head or shoulders touch the floor, or allowing the hips to come off the floor. If you allow the hips to raise off the floor and the head and shoulders to touch the floor, you will most likely "swing up" on the next sit-up, which minimizes the work of the abdominal muscles. If you cannot curl up with the arms on the chest, place the hands by the side of the hips or even help yourself up by holding on to your thighs (illustrations d and e). Do not perform the sit-up exercise with your legs completely extended, as this will cause strain on the lower back.

Muscles Developed:
Abdominal muscles and hip flexors.

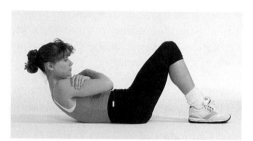

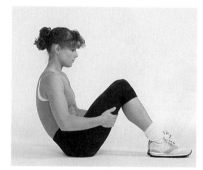

d   **e**

EXERCISE **5**

Leg Curl

Action: Lie on the floor face down. Cross the right ankle over the left heel. Apply resistance with your right foot, while you bring the left foot up to 90° at the knee joint. (Apply enough resistance so that the left foot can only be brought up slowly.) Repeat the exercise, crossing the left ankle over the right heel.

Muscles Developed: Hamstrings (and quadriceps).

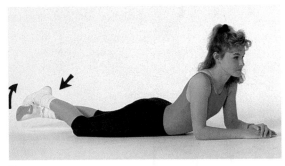

a

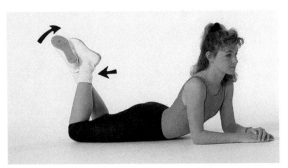

b

EXERCISE 6

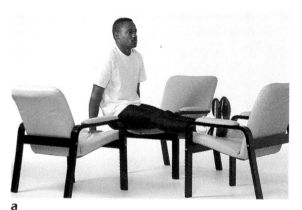

a

Modified Dip

Action: Place your hands and feet on opposite chairs with knees slightly bent (make sure that the chairs are well stabilized). Dip down at least to a 90° angle at the elbow joint, then return to the initial position. To increase the resistance, have someone else hold you down by the shoulders on the way up (see illustration c).

Muscles Developed:
Triceps, deltoid, and pectoralis major.

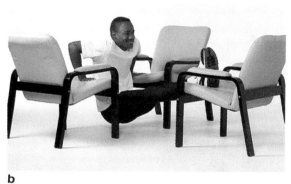

b

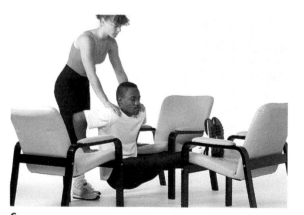

c

EXERCISE 7

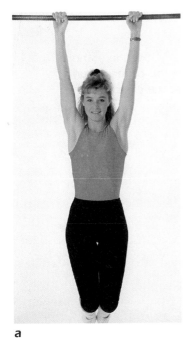

a

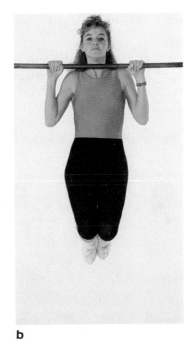

b

Pull-Up

Action: Suspend yourself from a bar with a pronated grip (thumbs in). Pull your body up until your chin is above the bar, then lower the body slowly to the starting position. If you are unable to perform the pull-up as described, either have a partner hold your feet to push off and facilitate the movement upward (illustrations c and d) or use a lower bar and support your feet on the floor (illustration e).

Muscles Developed: Biceps, brachioradialis, brachialis, trapezius, and latissimus dorsi.

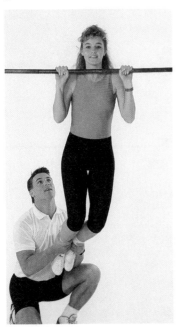

c

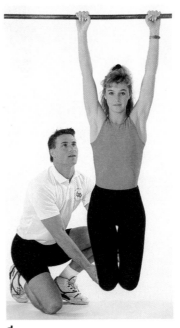

d

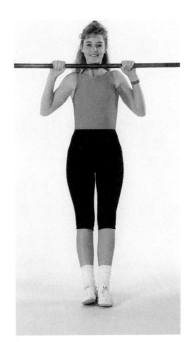

e

EXERCISE 8 ─────────────────────────────────

Arm Curl

Action: Using a palms-up grip, start with the arm completely extended, and with the aid of a sandbag or bucket filled (as needed) with sand or rocks, curl up as far as possible, then return to the initial position. Repeat the exercise with the other arm.

Muscles Developed: Biceps, brachioradialis, and brachialis.

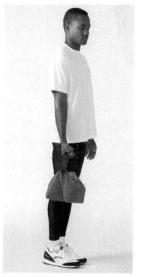 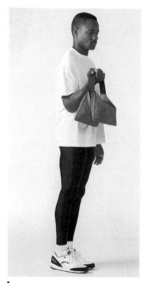

a   b

EXERCISE **9**

Heel Raise

Action: From a standing position with feet flat on the floor, raise and lower your body weight by moving at the ankle joint only (for added resistance, have someone else hold your shoulders down as you perform the exercise).

Muscles Developed: Gastrocnemius and soleus.

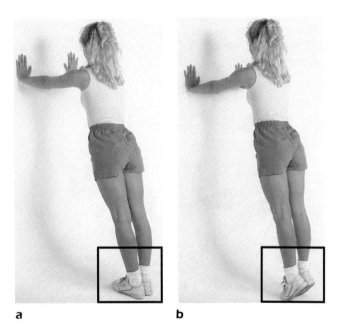

a   b

EXERCISE **10**

Leg Abduction and Adduction

Action: Both participants sit on the floor. The subject on the left places the feet on the inside of the other participant's feet. Simultaneously, the subject on the left presses the legs laterally (to the outside — abduction), while the subject on the right presses the legs medially (adduction). Hold the contraction for five to ten seconds. Repeat the exercise at all three angles, and then reverse the pressing sequence. The subject on the left places the feet on the outside and presses inward, while the subject on the right presses outward.

Muscles Developed: Hip abductors (rectus femoris, sartori, gluteus medius and minimus), and adductors (pectineus, gracilis, adductor magnus, adductor longus, and adductor brevis).

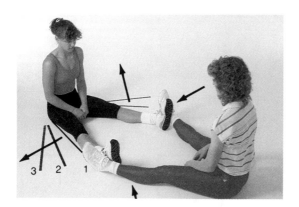

Strength-Training Exercises With Weights

EXERCISE **11**

Arm Curl

Action: Use a supinated or palms-up grip, and start with the arms almost completely extended. Now curl up as far as possible, then return to the starting position.

Muscles Developed: Biceps, brachioradialis, and brachialis.

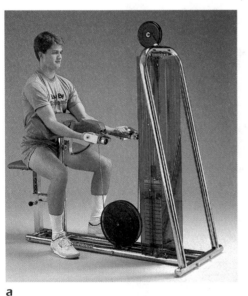

a

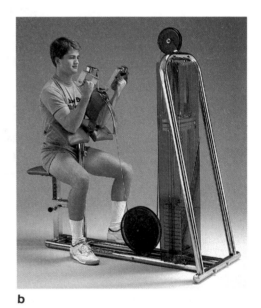

b

EXERCISE **12**

Bench Press

Action: Lie down on the bench with the head by the weight stack, the bench press bar above the chest, and keep the feet on the floor. Grasp the bar handles and press upward until the arms are completely extended, then return to the original position. Do not arch the back during this exercise.

Muscles Developed: Pectoralis major, triceps, and deltoid.

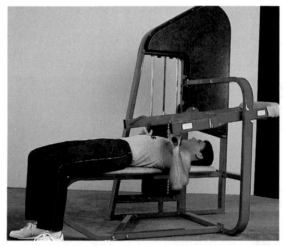

a

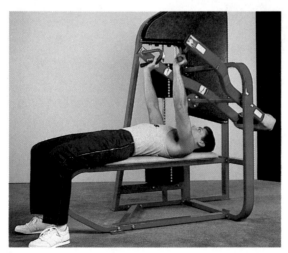

b

EXERCISE **13** ————————————————————————

Sit-Up

Action: Using either a horizontal or an inclined board, stabilize your feet and flex the knees to about 100 to 120°. Start with the head and shoulders off the board, curl all the way up, then return to the starting position without letting the head and shoulder touch the board (do not swing up, but rather curl up). You may curl straight up or use a twisting motion (twisting as you first start to come up), alternating on each sit-up.

Muscles Developed: Abdominals and hip flexors.

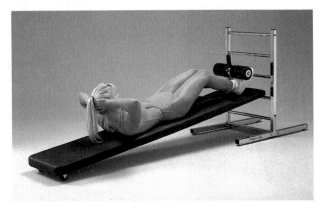

a

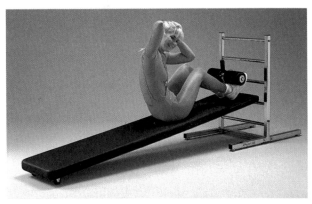

b

EXERCISE **14**

Leg Extension

Action: Sit in an upright position with the feet under the padded bar and grasp the handles at the sides. Extend the legs until they are completely straight, then return to the starting position.

Muscles Developed: Quadriceps.

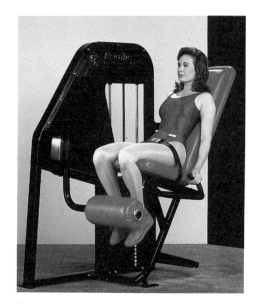

a

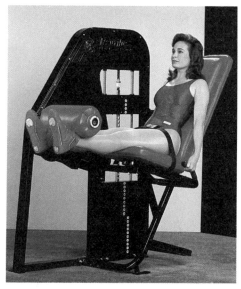

b

EXERCISE **15** _____

Leg Curl

Action: Lie with the face down on the bench, legs straight, and place the back of the feet under the padded bar. Curl up to at least 90°, and return to the original position.

Muscles Developed: Hamstrings.

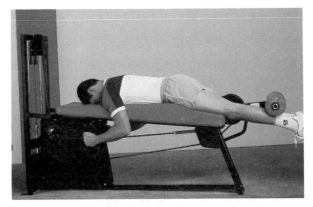

a

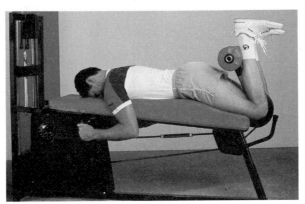

b

EXERCISE **16**

Lat Pull-Down

Action: Start from a sitting position, and hold the exercise bar with a wide grip. Pull the bar down until it touches the base of the neck, then return to the starting position (if a heavy resistance is used, stabilization of the body may be required by either using equipment as shown or by having someone else hold you down by the waist or shoulders).

Muscles Developed: Latissimus dorsi, pectoralis major, and biceps.

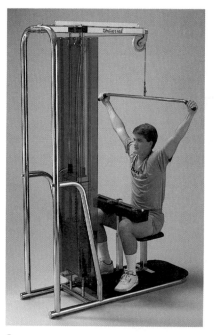

a

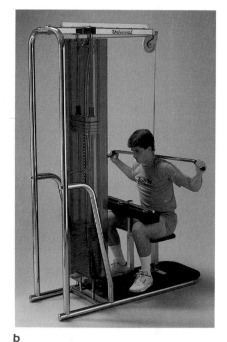

b

EXERCISE **17**

Heel Raise

Action: Start with your feet either flat on the floor or the front of the feet on an elevated block, then raise and lower yourself by moving at the ankle joint only. If additional resistance is needed, you can use a squat strength-training machine.

Muscles Developed: Gastrocnemius and soleus.

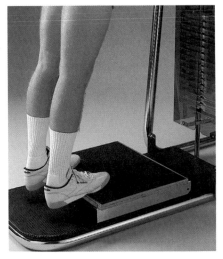
a

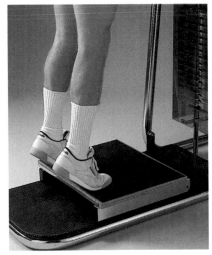
b

Flexibility Exercises

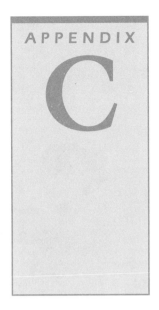

EXERCISE **18**

Lateral Head Tilt

Action: Slowly and gently tilt the head laterally. Repeat several times to each side.

Areas Stretched: Neck flexors and extensors and ligaments of the cervical spine.

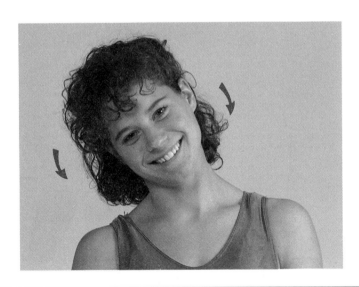

EXERCISE **19**

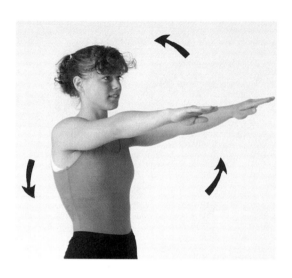

Arm Circles

Action: Gently circle your arms all the way around. Conduct the exercise in both directions.

Areas Stretched: Shoulder muscles and ligaments.

EXERCISE **20**

Side Stretch

Action: Stand straight up, feet separated to shoulder width, and place your hands on your waist. Now move the upper body to one side and hold the final stretch for a few seconds. Repeat on the other side.

Areas Stretched: Muscles and ligaments in the pelvic region.

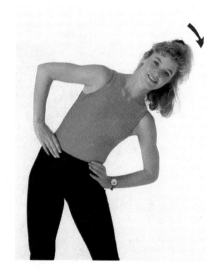

EXERCISE **21**

Body Rotation

Action: Place your arms slightly away from your body and rotate the trunk as far as possible, holding the final position for several seconds. Conduct the exercise for both the right and left sides of the body. You can also perform this exercise by standing about two feet away from the wall (back toward the wall), and then rotate the trunk, placing the hands against the wall.

Areas Stretched: Hip, abdominal, chest, back, neck, and shoulder muscles; hip and spinal ligaments.

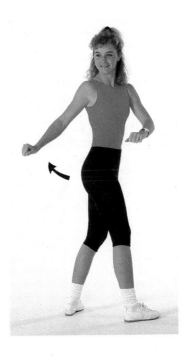

EXERCISE **22**

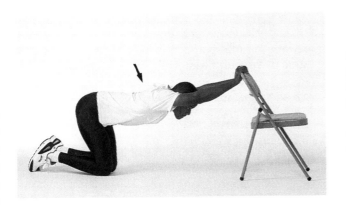

Chest Stretch

Action: Kneel down behind a chair and place both hands on the back of the chair. Gradually push your chest downward and hold for a few seconds.

Areas Stretched: Chest (pectoral) muscles and shoulder ligaments.

EXERCISE **23**

Shoulder Hyperextension Stretch

Action: Have a partner grasp your arms from behind by the wrists and slowly push them upward. Hold the final position for a few seconds.

Areas Stretched: Deltoid and pectoral muscles, and ligaments of the shoulder joint.

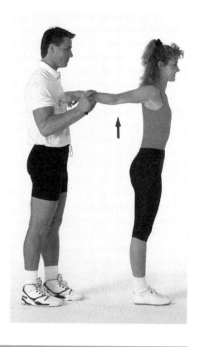

EXERCISE **24**

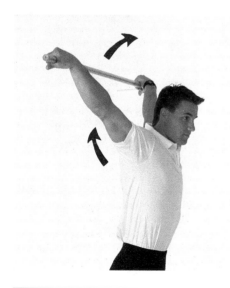

Shoulder Rotation Stretch

Action: With the aid of surgical tubing or an aluminum or wood stick, place the tubing or stick behind your back and grasp the two ends using a reverse (thumbs-out) grip. Slowly bring the tubing or stick over your head, keeping the elbows straight. Repeat several times (bring the hands closer together for additional stretch).

Areas Stretched: Deltoid, latissimus dorsi, and pectoral muscles; shoulder ligaments.

EXERCISE **25**

Quad Stretch

Action: Stand straight up and bring up one foot, flexing the knee. Grasp the front of the ankle and pull the ankle toward the gluteal region. Hold for several seconds. Repeat with the other leg.

Areas Stretched: Quadriceps muscle, and knee and ankle ligaments.

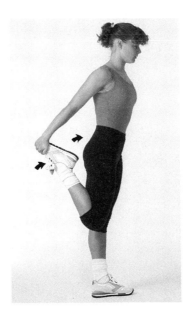

EXERCISE **26**

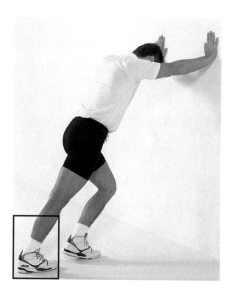

Heel Cord Stretch

Action: Stand against the wall or at the edge of a step and stretch the heel downward, alternating legs. Hold the stretched position for a few seconds.

Areas Stretched: Heel cord (Achilles tendon), gastrocnemius, and soleus muscles.

EXERCISE **27**

Adductor Stretch

Action: Stand with your feet about twice shoulder width and place your hands slightly above the knee. Flex one knee and slowly go down as far as possible, holding the final position for a few seconds. Repeat with the other leg.

Areas Stretched: Hip adductor muscles.

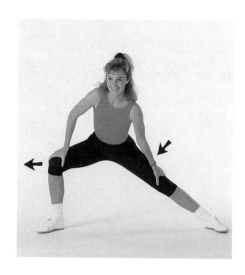

EXERCISE **28**

Sitting Adductor Stretch

Action: Sit on the floor and bring your feet in close to you, allowing the soles of the feet to touch each other. Now place your forearms (or elbows) on the inner part of the thigh and push the legs downward, holding the final stretch for several seconds.

Areas Stretched: Hip adductor muscles.

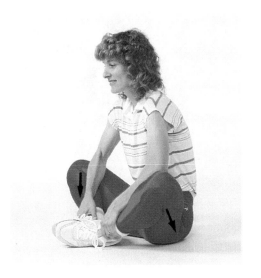

EXERCISE **29**

Sit-and-Reach Stretch

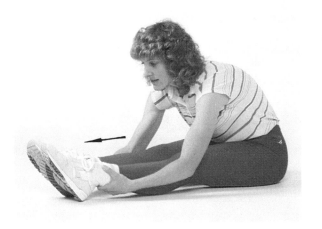

Action: Sit on the floor with legs together and gradually reach forward as far as possible. Hold the final position for a few seconds. This exercise may also be performed with the legs separated, reaching to each side as well as to the middle.

Areas Stretched: Hamstrings and lower back muscles, and lumbar spine ligaments.

Fitness and Wellness

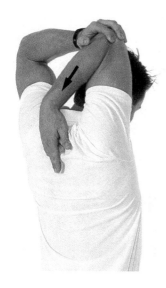

Triceps Stretch

Action: Place the right hand behind your neck. Grasp the right arm above the elbow with the left hand. Gently pull the elbow backward. Repeat the exercise with the opposite arm.

Areas Stretched: Back of upper arm (triceps muscle) and shoulder joint.

Exercises for the Prevention and Rehabilitation of Low Back Pain

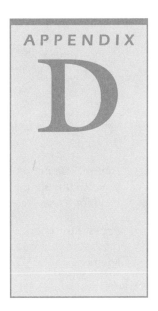

EXERCISE **31**

Single-Knee to Chest Stretch

Action: Lie down flat on the floor. Bend one leg at approximately 100° and gradually pull the opposite leg toward your chest. Hold the final stretch for a few seconds. Switch legs and repeat the exercise.

Areas Stretched: Lower back and hamstring muscles, and lumbar spine ligaments.

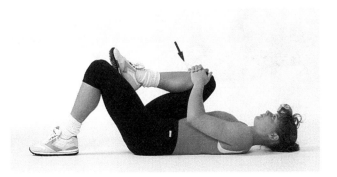

EXERCISE **32**

Double-Knee to Chest Stretch

Action: Lie flat on the floor and then slowly curl up into a fetal position. Hold for a few seconds.

Areas Stretched: Upper and lower back and hamstring muscles; spinal ligaments.

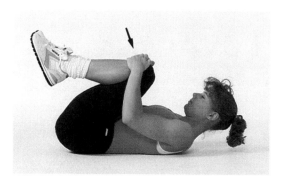

EXERCISE **33**

Upper and Lower Back Stretch

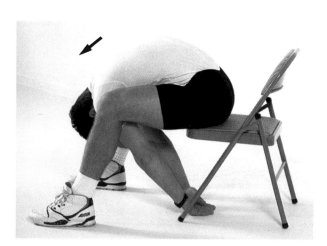

Action: Sit in a chair with feet separated greater than shoulder width. Place your arms to the inside of the thighs and bring your chest down toward the floor. At the same time, attempt to reach back as far as you can with your arms.

Areas Stretched: Upper and lower back muscles and ligaments.

EXERCISE **34** ──────────────────────────────

Sit-and-Reach Stretch

(see Exercise 29 in Appendix C)

EXERCISE **35** ──────────────────────────────

Side and Lower Back Stretch

Action: As illustrated in the photograph, sit on the floor with knees bent, feet to the right side, the left foot touching the right knee, and both legs flat on the floor. Place the right hand on the left knee and the left hand next to the right hand slightly above the knee. Gently pull the right shoulder toward the left knee and at the same time you may rotate the upper body counterclockwise. Switch sides and repeat the exercise (do not arch your back while performing this exercise).

Areas Stretched: Side and lower back muscles and lower back ligaments.

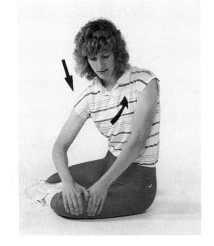

Note: The stretch is felt primarily when people experience low back pain due to muscle spasm or contracture.

EXERCISE **36**

Gluteal Stretch

Action: Sit on the floor, bend the right leg and place your right ankle slightly above the left knee. Grasp the left thigh with both hands and gently pull the leg toward your chest. Repeat the exercise with the opposite leg.

Areas Stretched: Buttock area (gluteal muscles).

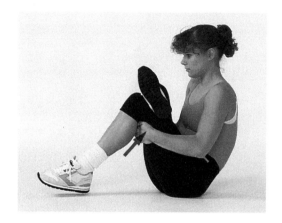

EXERCISE **37**

Trunk Rotation and Lower Back Stretch

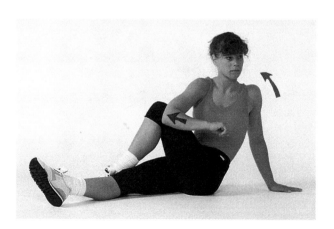

Action: Sit on the floor and bend the left leg, placing the left foot on the outside of the right knee. Place the right elbow on the left knee and push against it. At the same time, try to rotate the trunk to the left (counterclockwise). Hold the final position for a few seconds. Repeat the exercise with the other side.

Areas Stretched: Lateral side of the hip and thigh; trunk, and lower back.

EXERCISE 38

Pelvic Tilt

Action: Lie flat on the floor with the knees bent at about a 70° angle. Tilt the pelvis by tightening the abdominal muscles, flattening your back against the floor, and raising the lower gluteal area ever so slightly off the floor (see illustration b). Hold the final position for several seconds. The exercise can also be performed against a wall (as shown in illustration c).

Areas Stretched: Low back muscles and ligaments.

Areas Strengthened: Abdominal and gluteal muscles.

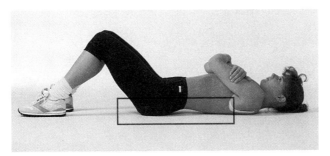

a

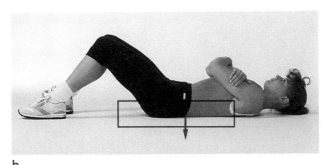

b

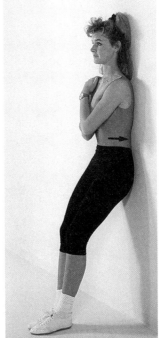

c

> **Note:** This is perhaps the most important exercise for the care of the lower back. It should be included as a part of the your daily exercise routine and should be performed several times throughout the day when pain in the lower back is present as a result of muscle imbalance.

EXERCISE **39** ————————————————————————

Abdominal Crunch and Abdominal Curl-Up

(see Exercise 4 in Appendix B)

It is important that you do not stabilize your feet when performing either of these exercises, because doing so decreases the work of the abdominal muscles. Also, remember not to "swing up" but rather to curl up as you perform these exercises.

Caloric, Protein, Fat, Saturated Fat, Cholesterol, and Carbohydrate Content of Selected Foods*

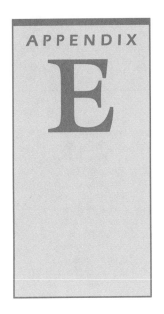

APPENDIX

E

Code	Food	Amount	Weight gm	Calories	Protein gm	Fat gm	Sat. Fat gm	Choles-terol mg	Carbo-hydrate gm
1.	Almond Joy, candy bar	1.5 oz.	42	227	2.5	12	10.2	0	28
2.	Almonds, shelled	1/4 c	36	213	6.6	19	1.4	0	9
3.	Apple, raw, unpared	1 med	150	80	0.3	1	0.0	0	20
4.	Apple juice, canned or bottled	1/2 c	124	59	0.1	0	0.0	0	15
5.	Applesauce, canned, sweetened	1/2 c	128	116	0.3	0	0.0	0	31
6.	Apricots, canned, heavy syrup	3 halves; 1¾ tbsp liq.	85	73	0.5	0	0.0	0	19
7.	Apricots, dried, sulfured, uncooked	10 med halves	35	91	1.8	0	0.0	0	23
8.	Apricots, raw	3 (12 per lb)	114	55	1.1	0	0.0	0	14
9.	Asparagus, cooked green spears	4 med	60	12	1.3	0	0.0	0	2
10.	Avocado, raw	1/2 med	120	185	2.4	19	3.2	0	7
11.	Bacon, cooked, drained	2 slices	15	86	3.8	8	2.7	30	1
12.	Bacon, lettuce, tomato sandwich	1	130	327	11.6	19	4.7	21	31
13.	Bagel	1 3½ in.	68	180	7.0	1	0.2	0	35
14.	Banana, raw	1 sm (7¼")	140	81	1.0	0	0.0	0	21
15.	Banana, nut bread	1 slice	50	169	3.0	8	1.5	33	22
16.	Beans, green snap, cooked	1/2 c	65	16	1.0	0	0.0	0	3
17.	Beans, lentils	1/4 c	50	53	3.9	0	0.0	0	10
18.	Beans, lima (Fordhook), froz., cooked	1/2 c	85	84	6.0	0	0.0	0	17
19.	Beans, red kidney, cooked	1 c	185	218	14.4	1	0.0	0	40
20.	Beans, refried	1/2 c	145	148	9.0	1	0.2	0	25
21.	Bean sprouts, mung, raw	1/2 c	52	18	2.0	0	0.0	0	4
22.	Beef, chuck, cooked,	3 oz.	85	212	25.0	12	7.8	80	0

*Reproduced with permission from Hoeger, W. W. K. Lifetime Physical Fitness & Wellness: A Personalized Program. Morton Publishing Company, 1992.

Code	Food	Amount	Weight gm	Calories	Protein gm	Fat gm	Sat. Fat gm	Choles- terol mg	Carbo- hydrate gm
23.	Beef, corned, canned	3 oz.	85	163	21.0	10	8.0	70	0
24.	Beef, ground, lean	3 oz.	85	186	23.3	10	5.0	81	0
25.	Beef, meatloaf	1 piece	111	246	20.0	15	6.1	125	6
26.	Beef, round steak, cooked, trimmed	3 oz.	85	222	24.3	13	6.0	77	0
27.	Beef, rump roast	3 oz.	85	177	24.7	9	4.0	80	0
28.	Beef, sirloin, cooked	3 oz.	85	329	19.6	27	13.0	77	0
29.	Beef, T-bone steak	3 oz.	85	403	16.7	37	15.6	66	0
30.	Beef, thin, sliced	3 oz.	85	105	18.5	3	1.4	36	0
31.	Beer	12 fl. oz.	360	151	1.1	0	1.1	0	14
32.	Beer, light	12 fl. oz.	354	96	0.7	0	0.0	0	4
33.	Beets, red, canned, drained	1/2 c	80	32	0.8	0	0.0	0	8
34.	Beet greens, cooked	1/2 c	73	13	1.3	0	0.0	0	2
35.	Biscuits, baking powder	1 med	35	114	2.5	6	1.1	0	18
36.	Blueberries, fresh cultivated	1/2 c	73	45	0.5	0	0.0	0	11
37.	Bologna	1 slice (1 oz.)	28	86	3.4	8	3.0	15	0
38.	Bologna, turkey	2 slices	57	113	7.8	9	3.0	56	1
39.	Bouillon, broth	1 cube	4	5	0.8	0	0.0	0	0
40.	Brandy	1 oz.	28	69	0.0	0	0.0	0	11
41.	Bread, Corn	1 slice	78	161	5.8	6	0.1	0	23
42.	Bread, Cracked wheat	1 slice	25	65	2.3	1	0.2	0	12
43.	Bread, French enriched	1 slice	35	102	3.2	1	0.2	0	19
44.	Bread, Oatmeal	1 slice	25	65	2.1	1	0.2	0	12
45.	Bread, Pita pocket	1 piece	60	165	6.2	1	0.1	0	33
46.	Bread, Pumpernickel	1 slice	32	80	2.9	1	0.2	0	15
47.	Bread, Rye (American)	1 slice	25	61	2.3	0	0.0	0	13
48.	Bread, white enriched	1 slice	25	68	2.2	1	0.2	0	13
49.	Bread, whole wheat	1 slice	25	61	2.6	1	0.6	0	12
50.	Broccoli, cooked drained	1 sm stalk	140	36	4.3	0	0.0	0	6
51.	Broccoli, raw	1 sm stalk	114	38	4.1	0	0.0	0	7
52.	Brownies, with nuts	1	20	95	1.3	6	2.3	18	11
53.	Brussels sprouts, froz., cooked, drained	1/2 c	78	28	3.2	0	0.0	0	5
54.	Bulgur, wheat	1 c	135	227	8.4	1	0.0	0	47
55.	Burrito, bean	1	166	307	12.5	9.5	3.6	14	45
56.	Burrito, combination, Taco Bell	1	175	404	21.0	16	0.0	0	43
57.	Butter	1 tsp	5	36	0.0	4	0.4	12	0
58.	Buttermilk, cultured	1 c	245	88	8.8	0	1.3	5	12
59.	Cabbage, boiled, drained wedge	1/2 c	85	16	0.9	0	0.0	0	3
60.	Cabbage, raw chopped	1/2 c	45	11	0.6	0	0.0	0	3
61.	Cake, Angel food, plain	1 piece	60	161	4.3	0	0.0	0	36
62.	Cake, Carrot	1 piece	96	385	4.2	21	4.1	74	48
63.	Cake, Cheesecake	1 piece (3½")	85	257	4.6	16	9.0	150	24
64.	Cake, Chocolate, w/icing	1 piece	69	235	3.0	8	3.6	37	40
65.	Cake, Coffee	1 piece	72	230	4.5	7	2.5	47	38
66.	Cake, Devil's food, iced	1 piece	99	365	4.5	16	5.0	68	55
67.	Cake, Pound	1 piece	30	120	2.0	5	1.0	32	15
68.	Cake, White, choc. icing	1 piece	71	268	3.5	11	3.7	2	48
69.	Candy, hard	1 oz.	28	109	0.0	0	0.0	0	28
70.	Cantaloupe	1/4 melon 5" diam.	239	35	2.0	0	0.0	0	10
71.	Caramel (candy, plain or choc.)	1 oz.	28	113	1.1	3	1.6	0	22

Code	Food	Amount	Weight gm	Calories	Protein gm	Fat gm	Sat. Fat gm	Choles- terol mg	Carbo- hydrate gm
72.	Carrots, cooked, drained	1/2 c	73	23	0.7	0	0.0	0	5
73.	Carrots, raw	1 carrot 7½" long	81	30	0.8	0	0.0	0	7
74.	Cashew, roasted, unsalted	2 oz.	57	326	9.2	27	5.4	0	16
75.	Cauliflower, cooked, drained	1/2 c	63	14	1.5	0	0.0	0	3
76.	Celery, green, raw, long	1 outer stalk 8"	40	7	0.4	0	0.0	0	2
77.	Cereal, All-Bran	1/4 c	21	53	3.0	0	0.1	0	16
78.	Cereal, Alpha Bits	1 c	28	111	2.2	1	0.0	0	25
79.	Cereal, Bran	1/2 c	30	72	3.8	1	0.0	0	22
80.	Cereal, Cheerios	1 c	23	89	3.4	1	1.2	0	16
81.	Cereal, Corn Chex	1 c	28	111	2.0	0	0.1	0	25
82.	Cereal, Corn Flakes	1 c	25	97	2.0	0	0.0	0	21
83.	Cereal, Cream of Wheat	1 c	244	140	3.6	1	0.1	0	29
84.	Cereal, Frosted Mini-Wheats	4 biscuits	31	111	3.2	0	0.0	0	26
85.	Cereal, Fruit & Fibre w/dates	1 c	56	180	6.0	2	0.3	0	42
86.	Cereal, Granola, Nature Valley	1/2 c	57	252	5.8	10	7.0	0	38
87.	Cereal, Grape Nuts	1/2 c	57	202	6.6	0	0.0	0	47
88.	Cereal, Life	1 c	44	162	8.1	1	0.1	0	32
89.	Cereal, Nutri-Grain Wheat	1 c	44	158	3.8	1	0.1	0	37
90.	Cereal, Oatmeal, quick, cooked	1/2 c	120	66	2.4	1	0.2	0	12
91.	Cereal, Raisin Bran	1 c	49	160	4.0	1	0.2	0	40
92.	Cereal, Rice Krispies	3/4 c	22	85	1.4	0	0.0	0	19
93.	Cereal, Shredded Wheat	1 c	19	65	2.1	0	0.0	0	11
94.	Cereal, Special K	1 c	21	83	4.2	0	0.0	0	16
95.	Cereal, Sugar Corn Pops	1 c	28	108	1.4	0	0.0	0	26
96.	Cereal, Sugar Frosted Flakes	1 c	35	133	1.8	0	0.0	0	32
97.	Cereal, Sugar Smacks	1 c	37	141	2.7	1	0.1	0	32
98.	Cereal, Total	1 c	33	116	3.3	1	0.1	0	26
99.	Cereal, Wheat Chex	1 c	46	169	4.5	1	0.2	0	38
100.	Cereal, whole wheat, cooked	1/2 c	123	55	2.2	0	0.0	0	12
101.	Cereal, whole wheat flakes, ready-to-eat	1 c	30	106	3.1	1	0.0	0	24
102.	Cereal, 40% Bran Flakes	1 c	39	125	4.9	1	0.1	0	31
103.	Cereal, 100% Bran	1/2 c	33	89	4.2	2	0.3	0	24
104.	Champagne	4 oz.	113	87	0.2	0	0.1	0	2
105.	Cheese, American	1 oz. slice	28	100	6.0	8	5.6	27	0
106.	Cheese, Bleu	1 oz.	28	100	6.0	8	5.3	25	1z
107.	Cheese, Cheddar	1 oz.	28	114	7.0	9	6.0	30	0
108.	Cheese, Cottage, 2%	1/2 c	113	103	15.5	2	1.4	10	4
109.	Cheese, Cottage, creamed	1/2 c	105	112	14.0	5	6.4	15	3
110.	Cheese, Creamed	1 oz.	28	99	6.0	8	3.0	31	1
111.	Cheese, Feta	1 oz.	28	75	4.5	6	4.2	25	1
112.	Cheese, Monterey jack	1 oz.	28	106	6.9	9	5.4	26	0
113.	Cheese, Mozzarella, skim	1 oz.	28	80	7.6	5	3.1	15	1
114.	Cheese, Parmesan	1 tbsp	5	23	2.1	2	1.0	4	0
115.	Cheese, Ricotta, part skim	1 oz.	28	39	3.2	2	1.4	9	1
116.	Cheese, Souffle	1 portion	110	240	10.9	19	9.5	189	7
117.	Cheese, Swiss	1 oz.	28	107	8.0	8	5.0	26	1
118.	Cheese puffs, Cheetos	1 oz.	28	158	2.2	10	4.8	5	14
119.	Cheeseburger, McDonald's	1	115	321	15.2	16	6.7	40	29
120.	Cherries	10	75	47	0.9	0	0.0	0	12
121.	Chicken, BK Broiler sandwich, Burger King	1 sandwich	168	379	24.0	18	3.0	53	31

Code	Food	Amount	Weight gm	Calories	Protein gm	Fat gm	Sat. Fat gm	Choles- terol mg	Carbo- hydrate gm
122.	Chicken breast, roast w/skin	1	98	193	29.2	8	2.1	83	0
123.	Chicken chow mein	1 c	250	255	31.0	11	3.6	75	10
124.	Chicken, drumstick Kentucky Fried	1	54	136	14.0	8	2.2	73	2
125.	Chicken, drumstick, roasted	1	52	112	14.1	6	1.6	48	0
126.	Chicken McNuggets	6	111	329	19.5	21	5.2	64	15
127.	Chicken, patty sandwich	1	157	436	24.8	23	6.1	68	34
128.	Chicken, wing, Kentucky Fried	1	45	151	11.0	10	2.9	70	4
129.	Chicken, roast, light meat without skin	3 oz.	85	141	27.0	3	0.4	45	0
130.	Chicken, roast, dark meat without skin	3 oz.	85	149	24.0	5	0.8	50	0
131.	Chili con carne	1 c	255	339	19.1	16	5.8	28	31
132.	Chocolate fudge	1 oz.	28	115	0.6	3	2.1	1	21
133.	Chocolate, milk	1 oz.	28	147	2.0	9	3.6	5	16
134.	Chocolate, milk w/almonds	1 oz.	28	150	2.9	10	4.4	5	15
135.	Clam, canned, drained	3 oz.	85	83	13.0	2	0.2	50	2
136.	Cocoa, hot, with whole milk	1 c	250	218	9.1	9	6.1	33	26
137.	Cocoa, plain, dry	1 tbsp	5	14	0.9	1	0.0	0	3
138.	Coconut, shredded, packed	1/2 c	65	225	2.3	23	20.0	0	6
139.	Cod, batter fried	3.5 oz.	100	199	19.6	10	3.9	55	8
140.	Cod, cooked	3 oz.	85	144	24.3	4	1.5	60	0
141.	Cod, poached	3.5 oz.	100	94	20.9	1	0.3	60	0
142.	Coffee	3/4 cup	180	1	0.0	0	0.0	0	0
143.	Coleslaw	1 c	120	173	1.6	17	1.0	5	6
144.	Collards, leaves without stems, cooked, drained	1/2 c	95	32	3.4	1	2.0	0	5
145.	Cookies, Chocolate chip homemade	2 2¼" diam.	20	103	1.0	6	1.7	14	12
146.	Cookies, Fig bars	4 bars	56	210	2.0	4	1.0	27	42
147.	Cookies, Oatmeal raisin	2 2" diam.	26	122	1.5	5	1.3	1	18
148.	Cookies, Peanut butter, homemade	2 cookies	24	123	2.0	7	2.0	11	14
149.	Cookies, sandwich, all	4 cookies	40	195	2.0	8	2.0	0	29
150.	Cookies, Shortbread	4 cookies	32	155	2.0	8	2.9	27	20
151.	Cookies, Vanilla	5 1¾" diam.	20	93	1.0	3	0.8	10	15
152.	Cookies, Vanilla wafers	10 wafers	40	185	2.0	7	1.8	25	29
153.	Corn, boiled on cob	1 ear 5" long	140	70	2.5	1	0.0	0	16
154.	Corn, canned, drained	1/2 c	83	70	2.2	1	0.0	0	16
155.	Corn chips	1 oz.	28	155	2.0	9	1.8	0	16
156.	Cornmeal, degermed, yellow, enriched, cooked	1/2 c	120	60	1.3	0	0.0	0	13
157.	Crab, canned	1 c	135	135	23.0	3	0.5	135	1
158.	Crackers, Cheese	10 crackers	10	50	1.0	3	0.9	6	5
159.	Crackers, Graham	2 squares	14	55	1.1	1	0.3	0	10
160.	Crackers, Ritz	1 cracker	3	15	0.2	1	0.2	0	2
161.	Crackers, Ryewafers, whole grain	2 crackers	14	55	1.0	1	0.3	0	10
162.	Crackers, Saltines	4 squares	11	48	1.0	1	0.3	0	8
163.	Crackers, Soda	1	3	13	0.3	0	0.1	0	2
164.	Crackers, Triscuits	1	5	23	0.4	1	0.3	0	3
165.	Crackers, Wheat Thins	1	2	9	0.2	0	0.1	0	1
166.	Cranberry juice	1 c	253	145	0.1	0	0.0	0	36

Code	Food	Amount	Weight gm	Calories	Protein gm	Fat gm	Sat. Fat gm	Choles-terol mg	Carbo-hydrate gm
167.	Cream, light coffee or table	1 tbsp	15	20	0.5	2	0.5	5	1
168.	Cream, heavy whipping	1 tbsp	15	53	0.3	6	1.3	12	1
169.	Croissant	1	57	235	4.7	12	4.0	13	27
170.	Croissants (Sara Lee)	1 roll	18	59	1.6	2	0.3	0	8
171.	Croissan'wich, egg, cheese Burger King	1 sandwich	110	315	13.0	20	7.0	222	19
172.	Cucumbers, raw pared	9 sm slices	28	4	0.3	0	0.0	0	1
173.	Dates hydrated	5	46	110	0.9	0	0.0	0	29
174.	Doughnut, plain	1	42	164	1.9	8	2.0	19	22
175.	Doughnut, yeast raised	1	27	235	4.0	13	5.2	21	26
176.	Dressing, Bleu cheese	1 tbsp	15	77	0.7	8	1.9	4	1
177.	Dressing, French	1 tbsp	16	83	0.1	9	1.4	0	1
178.	Dressing, French, low cal	1 tbsp.	15	24	0.0	2	0.2	0	2
179.	Dressing, Italian	1 tbsp.	15	69	0.1	9	1.3	0	2
180.	Dressing, Italian, low cal	1 tbsp.	15	10	0.0	1	0.0	0	1
181.	Dressing, Ranch style	1 tbsp.	15	54	0.4	6	0.9	6	1
182.	Dressing, Thousand island	1 tbsp.	15	60	0.2	6	1.0	4	2
183.	Dressing, Thousand island, low cal	1 tbsp.	15	25	0.1	2	0.2	2	3
184.	Eggs, hard cooked	1 large	50	72	6.0	5	1.8	250	1
185.	Egg, fried with butter	1	46	95	5.4	6	2.4	278	1
186.	Egg McMuffin	1	138	327	18.5	15	5.9	259	31
187.	Egg salad sandwich	1	111	325	10.0	19	3.9	215	28
188.	Egg, scrambled, with milk, butter	1 egg	64	95	6.0	7	3.0	282	1
189.	Eggs, white	1 large	33	17	3.6	0	0.0	0	0
190.	Eggs, yolk, raw	1 yolk	17	63	2.8	6	1.7	248	0
191.	Enchilada, beef	1	200	487	21.8	23	8.8	63	26
192.	Enchilada, cheese	1	230	632	25.3	34	17.6	82	31
193.	Figs, dried	1 large	21	60	1.0	0	0.0	0	15
194.	Filet of Fish, McDonald's	1	131	402	15.0	23	7.9	43	34
195.	Fish, sticks	2	56	140	12.0	6	1.6	52	8
196.	Flounder	3 oz.	85	171	25.5	7	1.0	60	0
197.	Flour, all purpose enriched	1 c	125	455	13.0	1	0.0	0	95
198.	Flour, whole wheat	1 c	120	400	16.0	2	0.0	0	85
199.	Frankfurter, cooked	1	57	176	7.0	16	5.6	45	1
200.	Frankfurter, turkey, cooked	1	45	102	6.4	8	2.7	39	1
201.	French toast	1 piece	65	123	4.9	4	1.1	73	15
202.	Fruit cocktail	1 c	245	91	1.0	0	0.0	0	24
203.	Fruit cocktail, juice pack	1 c	248	115	1.1	0	0.0	0	29
204.	Grapefruit, raw white	1/2 med	301	56	1.0	0	0.0	0	15
205.	Grapefruit, juice unsweetened canned	1/2 c	124	50	0.6	0	0.0	0	12
206.	Grapes, seedless, European	10 grapes	50	34	0.3	0	0.0	0	9
207.	Grape juice, unsweetened bottled	1/2 c	127	84	0.3	0	0.0	0	21
208.	Gravy, beef, homemade	1 tbsp	17	19	0.3	2	1.0	1	1
209.	Haddock, fried (dipped in egg, milk, bread crumbs)	3 oz.	85	141	17.0	5	1.0	54	5
210.	Halibut, broiled with butter or margarine	3 oz.	85	144	21.0	6	2.1	55	0
211.	Ham (cured pork)	3 oz.	85	318	20.0	26	9.4	77	0
212.	Ham, lunch meat	1 slice	28	37	5.5	1	0.5	13	.3
213.	Hamburger, Big Mac	1	204	581	25.1	36	12.0	85	40
214.	Hamburger bun	1 bun	40	129	3.7	2	1.0	0	23

Fitness and Wellness

Code	Food	Amount	Weight gm	Calories	Protein gm	Fat gm	Sat. Fat gm	Choles- terol mg	Carbo- hydrate gm
215.	Hamburger, McDonald's	1	99	257	13.0	9	3.7	26	30
216.	Hamburger, Quarter pounder	1 burger	160	427	24.6	24	9.1	80	29
217.	Hamburger, Quarter pounder, with cheese	1 burger	186	525	29.6	32	12.8	107	31
218.	Honey	1 tbsp	21	64	0.0	0	0.0	0	17
219.	Honeydew melon	1 slice (1/10 melon)	129	45	0.6	0	0.0	0	12
220.	Hotdog bun	1 bun	40	115	3.3	2	1.0	0	20
221.	Ice cream, vanilla	1/2 c	67	135	3.0	7	4.4	27	14
222.	Ice cream cone	1 small	115	185	4.3	5	2.2	24	30
223.	Ice cream cone, Dairy Queen	medium	142	230	6.0	7	4.6	15	35
224.	Ice cream, hot fudge sundae	1	164	357	7.0	11	5.4	27	58
225.	Ice milk, vanilla	1/2 c	61	100	3.0	3	1.8	13	15
226.	Instant breakfast, whole milk	1 c	281	280	15.0	8	5.1	33	34
227.	Instant breakfast, skim milk	1 c	282	216	15.4	0	0.0	4	35
228.	Jams or preserves	1 tbsp	7	18	0.0	0	0.0	0	5
229.	Jelly	1 tbsp	18	49	0.0	0	0.0	0	13
230.	Kale, fresh cooked, drained	1/2 c	55	22	2.5	0	0.0	0	3
231.	Kiwi fruit, raw	1 med	76	46	1.0	0	0.0	0	11
232.	Kool Aid, with sugar	1 c	240	100	0.0	0	0.0	0	25
233.	Lamb leg, roast, trimmed	3 oz.	85	237	22.0	16	7.3	60	0
234.	Lamb loin chop, broiled, lean	3 oz.	84	183	25.0	8	3.4	78	0
235.	Lasagna, homemade	1 piece	220	357	23.6	18	8.3	50	27
236.	Lemon juice, fresh	1 tbsp	15	4	0.1	0	0.0	0	1
237.	Lemonade (concentrate)	12 oz.	340	137	0.2	0	0.1	0	36
238.	Lentils, cooked	1/2 c	100	106	8.0	0	0.0	0	19
239.	Lettuce, crisp head	1 c sm chunks	75	10	0.7	0	0.0	0	2
240.	Lettuce, cos or romaine	1 c chopped	55	10	0.7	0	0.0	0	2
241.	Liver, beef, fried	1 slice 3 oz.	85	195	22.0	9	2.5	345	5
242.	Liverwurst, fresh	1 slice 1 oz.	28	87	5.0	7	3.5	50	1
243.	Lobster	1 c	145	138	27.0	2	1.0	293	0
244.	M&M's, Chocolate, plain	1 oz.	28	140	1.9	6	3.3	0	19
245.	M&M's, Chocolate, w/peanuts	1 oz.	28	145	3.2	7	3.2	0	17
246.	Macaroni, enriched, cooked	1/2 c	70	78	2.4	0	0.0	0	16
247.	Macaroni and cheese	1/2 c	100	215	8.2	11	4.0	21	20
248.	Margarine	1 tsp	5	34	0.0	4	0.7	2	0
249.	Mars bar	1 bar	50	240	4.0	11	4.8	0	30
250.	Matzo	1 piece	30	117	3.0	0	0.0	0	25
251.	Mayonnaise	1 tsp	5	36	0.0	4	0.7	3	0
252.	Milk, chocolate, 2%	1 c	250	180	8.0	5	3.1	17	26
253.	Milk, evaporated whole	1/2 c	126	172	9.0	10	5.8	40	13
254.	Milk, lowfat (2% fat)	1 c	246	145	10.0	5	3.1	5	15
255.	Milk shake, chocolate	1 (10 fluid oz.)	340	433	11.5	13	7.8	45	70
256.	Milk shake, strawberry	1 (10 fluid oz.)	340	383	11.4	10	6.0	37	64
257.	Milk shake, vanilla, McDonald's	1	289	323	10.0	8	5.1	29	52
258.	Milk, skim	1 c	245	88	9.0	0	0.3	5	12
259.	Milk, whole (3.5% fat)	1 c	244	159	9.0	9	5.1	34	12
260.	Milky Way bar	1 bar	60	260	3.2	9	5.4	14	43
261.	Molasses, medium	1 tbsp	20	50	0.0	0	0.0	0	13
262.	Muffin, blueberry	1	45	135	3.0	5	1.5	19	20
263.	Muffin, bran	1	45	125	3.0	6	1.4	24	19
264.	Muffin, cornmeal	1	45	145	3.0	5	1.5	23	21
265.	Muffin, English, plain	1	57	140	4.5	1	0.3	0	26
266.	Muffin, English w/butter	1	63	186	5.0	5	2.3	15	30

Content of Selected Food

Code	Food	Amount	Weight gm	Calories	Protein gm	Fat gm	Sat. Fat gm	Choles- terol mg	Carbo- hydrate gm
267.	Mushrooms, fresh cultivated	1/2 c sliced	35	12	1.0	0	0.0	0	2
268.	Mustard greens, cooked drained	1/2 c	70	16	1.7	0	0.0	0	3
269.	Noodles, egg, enriched cooked	1/2 c	80	100	3.3	1	0.0	0	19
270.	Nuts, Brazil	1 oz. (6-8 nuts)	28	185	4.1	19	4.8	0	3
271.	Nuts, Pecans	1 oz.	28	195	2.6	20	1.4	0	4
272.	Nuts, Walnuts	1 oz. (14 halves)	28	185	4.2	18	1.0	0	5
273.	Oil, Corn	1 tbsp.	15	125	0.0	14	1.8	0	0
274.	Oil, Olive	1 tbsp.	15	125	0.0	14	1.9	0	0
275.	Oil, Safflower	1 tbsp.	15	125	0.0	14	1.3	0	0
276.	Oil, Soybean	1 tsp.	5	44	0.0	5	2.0	0	0
277.	Okra, cooked, drained	1/2 c	80	23	1.6	0	0.0	0	5
278.	Olives, black, ripe	10 extra large	55	61	0.5	7	1.0	0	1
279.	Onions, mature, cooked, drained	1/2 c sliced	105	31	1.3	0	0.0	0	7
280.	Onion rings, fried	3	30	122	1.6	8	2.3	0	11
281.	Onion rings (Brazier) Dairy Queen	1 serving	85	360	6.0	17	6.0	15	33
282.	Orange juice, froz. reconstituted	1/2 c	125	61	0.9	0	0.0	0	15
283.	Orange, raw (medium skin)	1 med	180	64	1.3	0	0.0	0	16
284.	Oysters, Eastern, breaded, fried	1 oyster	45	90	5.0	5	1.4	35	5
285.	Oysters, raw, Eastern	1/2 c (6-9 med)	120	79	10.0	2	1.3	60	4
286.	Pancakes	1 6" diam x 1/2" thick	73	169	5.2	5	1.0	36	25
287.	Pancakes, buckwheat	1 4 in. diam.	27	55	2.0	2	0.9	20	6
288.	Pancakes w/butter, syrup	1 large	100	250	4.0	5	1.9	24	47
289.	Papaya, raw	1/2 med	227	60	0.9	0	0.0	0	15
290.	Parsnips, cooked	1 large 9" long	160	106	2.4	1	0.0	0	24
291.	Peaches, canned, heavy syrup	1 half 2⅛ tbsp liq.	96	75	0.4	0	0.0	0	19
292.	Peaches, canned, juice pack	1 half	77	34	0.5	0	0.0	0	9
293.	Peaches, raw, peeled	1 2¾" diam.	175	58	0.9	0	0.0	0	15
294.	Peanut butter	2 tbsp	32	188	8.0	16	1.0	0	6
295.	Peanut butter, jam sandwich	1	100	340	11.4	14	2.6	0	45
296.	Peanuts, roasted	1 oz.	28	166	7.0	14	1.0	0	5
297.	Pears, canned, heavy syrup	1 half 2¼ tbsp liq.	103	78	0.2	0	0.0	0	20
298.	Pears, canned, juice pack	1 half	77	38	0.3	0	0.0	0	10
299.	Pears, raw	1 pear	180	100	1.1	1	0.0	0	25
300.	Peas, canned, drained	1/2 c	85	75	4.0	0	0.0	0	14
301.	Peas, frozen, cooked drained	1/2 c	80	55	4.1	0	0.0	0	10
302.	Peppers, sweet, raw	1 pepper 3¼" x 3" diam.	200	36	2.0	0	0.0	0	8
303.	Pickles, dill	1 large 4" long	135	15	0.9	0	0.0	0	3
304.	Pickles, sweet	1 large 3" long	35	51	0.2	0	0.0	0	13
305.	Pie, Apple	1 piece (3½")	118	302	2.6	13	3.5	120	45
306.	Pie, Apple, fried	1 pie	85	255	2.2	14	5.8	14	32
307.	Pie, Blueberry	1 piece (3½")	158	380	4.0	17	4.0	0	55
308.	Pie, Cherry	1 piece (3½")	118	308	3.1	13	5.0	137	45
309.	Pie, Cherry, fried	1 pie	85	250	2.0	14	5.8	13	32
310.	Pie, Chocolate cream	1 piece (1/6 pie)	175	311	7.4	13	4.5	15	42
311.	Pie, Lemon meringue	1 piece (1/6 pie)	140	355	4.7	14	3.5	137	53
312.	Pie, Pecan	1 piece (1/6 pie)	138	583	6.3	24	3.9	13	92

Code	Food	Amount	Weight gm	Calories	Protein gm	Fat gm	Sat. Fat gm	Choles-terol mg	Carbo-hydrate gm
313.	Pie, Pumpkin	1 (3½")	114	241	4.6	13	3.0	70	28
314.	Pineapple, canned, heavy syrup	1/2 c	128	95	0.4	0	0.0	0	25
315.	Pineapple, canned, juice pack	1/2 c	125	75	0.5	0	0.0	0	20
316.	Pineapple, raw	1/2 c diced	78	41	0.3	0	0.0	0	11
317.	Pizza, Cheese, Thin 'n Crispy, Pizza Hut	1/2 10" pie	*	450	25.0	15	7.0	125	54
318.	Pizza, Cheese, Thick 'n Chewy, Pizza Hut	1/2 10" pie	*	560	34.0	14	6.0	110	71
319.	Plums, Japanese and hybrid, raw	1 plum 2⅛" diam.	70	32	0.3	0	0.0	0	8
320.	Popcorn, cooked, oil	1 c	11	55	0.9	3	0.5	0	6
321.	Popcorn, popped, plain, large kernel	1 c	6	12	0.8	0	0.0	0	5
322.	Pork, roast, trimmed	2 slices 3 oz.	85	179	24.0	8	2.2	65	0
323.	Pork, sausage, cooked	1 sm link	17	72	2.8	6	2.1	13	1
324.	Potato, au gratin	1 c	245	228	5.6	10	6.3	12	32
325.	Potato, baked in skin	1 potato 2⅓ x 4¼"	202	145	4.0	0	0.0	0	33
326.	Potato chips	10 chips	20	114	1.1	8	2.1	0	10
327.	Potato, French fried long	10 strips 3½-4"	78	214	3.4	10	1.7	0	28
328.	Potato, Hashbrowns, McDonald's	1 patty	55	144	1.4	9	3.0	4	15
329.	Potato, mashed, milk added	1/2 c	105	69	2.2	1	0.4	8	14
330.	Potato salad w/eggs, mayo	1/2 c	125	179	3.4	10	7.8	85	14
331.	Potato, hash brown	1/2 c	78	170	2.5	9	3.5	0	22
332.	Pretzel, thin, twists	1 oz.	28	113	2.8	1	0.3	0	23
333.	Prunes, dried "softenized" without pits	5 prunes	61	137	1.1	0	0.0	0	36
334.	Prune juice, canned or bottled	1/2 c	128	99	0.5	0	0.0	0	24
335.	Pudding, Chocolate, canned	5 oz.	142	205	3.0	11	9.5	1	30
336.	Pudding, Tapioca, canned	5 oz.	142	160	3.0	5	4.8	1	28
337.	Pudding, Vanilla, canned	5 oz.	142	220	2.0	10	9.5	1	33
338.	Quiche, Lorraine	1 piece	242	825	18.0	66	31.9	392	40
339.	Raisins, unbleached, seedless	1 oz.	28	82	0.7	0	0.0	0	22
340.	Raspberries, fresh	1 c	123	60	1.1	1	0.0	0	14
341.	Raspberries, frozen	1 c	250	255	1.7	1	0.0	0	62
342.	Rice, brown, cooked	1/2 c	96	116	2.5	1	0.0	0	25
343.	Rice, white enriched, cooked	1/2 c	103	113	2.1	0	0.0	0	25
344.	Rice, wild, cooked	1/2 c	100	92	3.6	0	0.0	0	19
345.	Roll, hard, white	1 roll	50	155	5.0	2	0.0	0	30
346.	Rueben sandwich	1	237	488	28.7	28	10.4	85	30
347.	Salad, Chef, Burger King	1 serving	273	178	17.0	9	4.0	103	7
348.	Salad, Chicken, Burger King	1 serving	258	142	20.0	4	1.0	49	8
349.	Salad, Chicken w/celery	1/2 c	78	266	10.5	25	4.1	48	1
350.	Salad, Tuna	1 c	205	375	33.0	19	3.3	80	19
351.	Salami, dry	1 oz.	28	128	7.0	11	1.6	24	0
352.	Salmon, broiled with butter or margarine	3 oz.	85	156	23.0	6	2.2	53	0
353.	Salmon, canned Chinook	3 oz.	85	179	16.6	12	0.8	30	0
354.	Sardines, canned drained	1 oz.	28	58	7.0	3	1.0	20	0
355.	Sauerkraut, canned	1/2 c	118	21	1.2	0	0.0	0	5
356.	Scallops, breaded, cooked	6 pieces	90	195	15.0	10	2.5	70	10
357.	Sherbet	1/2 c	97	135	1.1	2	1.3	7	29
358.	Shrimp, boiled	3 oz.	85	99	18.0	1	0.1	128	1
359.	Shrimp, fried	7 medium	85	200	16.0	10	2.5	168	11

Code	Food	Amount	Weight gm	Calories	Protein gm	Fat gm	Sat. Fat gm	Choles- terol mg	Carbo- hydrate gm
360.	Snickers bar	1 bar	61	290	6.6	4	5.4	0	37
361.	Soda pop, cola	12 oz.	369	144	0.0	0	0.0	0	37
362.	Soda pop, diet	12 oz.	340	2	0.1	0	0.0	0	0
363.	Soda pop, Ginger ale	12 oz.	366	113	0.0	0	0.0	0	29
364.	Soda pop, Lemon-lime	12 oz.	340	138	0.0	0	0.0	0	35
365.	Soda pop, Root beer	12 oz.	340	140	0.0	0	0.0	0	36
366.	Soup, Chicken, cream	1 c	248	191	7.5	12	4.6	27	15
367.	Soup, Chicken noodle	1 c	241	75	4.0	2	0.7	7	9
368.	Soup, Clam chowder, Manhattan	1 c	244	78	4.2	2	0.4	2	12
369.	Soup, Clam chowder, north east	1 c	248	163	9.5	7	3.0	22	16
370.	Soup, Cream of mushroom condensed, prepared with equal volume of milk	1 c	245	216	7.0	14	5.4	15	16
371.	Soup, Minestrone	1 c	241	80	4.3	3	0.5	2	11
372.	Soup, Split pea, condensed, prepared with equal volume of water	1 c	245	145	9.0	3	1.1	0	21
373.	Soup, Tomato, condensed, prepared with equal volume of water	1 c	245	88	2.0	3	0.5	0	16
374.	Soup, Tomato with milk	1 c	248	160	6.0	6	2.9	17	22
375.	Soup, vegetable beef, condensed, prepared with equal volume of water	1 c	245	78	5.0	2	0.0	0	10
376.	Soup, Vegetarian vegetable	1 c	250	70	2.1	2	0.3	0	12
377.	Sour cream	1 tbsp	14	30	0.4	3	1.8	6	1
378.	Soup cream, imitation	1 tbsp.	14	29	0.3	3	2.5	0	1
379.	Spaghetti, in tomato sauce with cheese	1 c	250	260	8.8	9	2.0	10	37
380.	Spaghetti, plain, cooked	1 c	140	155	5.0	1	0.1	0	32
381.	Spaghetti, whole wheat, cooked	1 c	125	151	6.6	1	0.1	0	32
382.	Spaghetti, with meatballs and tomato sauce	1 c	248	332	18.6	11.7	3.0	75	3
383.	Spareribs, cooked	3 oz.	85	377	17.8	33	12.0	73	0
384.	Spinach, canned, drained	1/2 c	103	25	2.3	1	0.0	0	4
385.	Spinach, froz., cooked, drained	1/2 c	103	24	3.1	0	0.0	0	4
386.	Spinach, raw, chopped	1 c	55	14	1.8	0	0.0	0	2
387.	Squash, summer, cooked	1/2 c	90	13	0.8	0	0.0	0	3
388.	Squash, winter, baked mashed	1/2 c	103	70	1.9	0	0.0	0	18
389.	Strawberries, frozen, sweetened	1 c	250	245	1.4	0	0.0	0	66
390.	Strawberries, raw	1 c	149	55	1.0	1	0.0	0	13
391.	Stuffing, bread, prepared	1/2 c	70	250	4.6	15	3.1	0	25
392.	Sundae, choc. Dairy Queen	medium	184	300	6.0	7	4.9	79	53
393.	Sugar, brown granulated	1 tsp	5	17	0.0	0	0.0	0	5
394.	Sugar, white granulated	1 tsp	4	15	0.0	0	0.0	0	4
395.	Sweet potato, baked	1 potato 5" long	146	161	2.4	1	0.0	0	37
396.	Syrup (maple)	1 tbsp	20	50	0.0	0	0.0	0	13
397.	Taco shell	1 shell	10	60	1.1	3	0.3	0	9
398.	Taco, Taco Bell	1	83	186	15.0	8	0.0	0	14
399.	Tangerine	1 med 2⅛" diam.	116	39	0.7	0	0.0	0	10
400.	Tartar sauce	1 tbsp.	14	74	0.2	8	1.2	4	1
401.	Tea, brewed	1/4 c	180	0	0.0	0	0.0	0	0

Code	Food	Amount	Weight gm	Calories	Protein gm	Fat gm	Sat. Fat gm	Choles- terol mg	Carbo- hydrate gm
402.	Tomato juice, canned	1 c	244	42	1.9	0	0.1	0	10
403.	Tomato sauce (catsup)	1 tbsp	15	16	0.3	0	0.0	0	4
404.	Tomato, canned	1/2 c	121	26	1.2	0	0.0	0	5
405.	Tomato, raw	1 tomato 3½ oz.	100	20	1.0	0	0.0	0	4
406.	Tortilla chips	1 oz.	28	139	2.2	8	1.1	0	17
407.	Tortilla, corn, lime	1 6" diam.	30	63	1.5	1	0.0	0	14
408.	Tortilla, flour	1	35	105	2.6	3	0.4	0	19
409.	Tostada	1	148	206	9.2	18	3.0	14	25
410.	Trout, broiled w/butter, lemon	3 oz.	85	175	21.0	9	4.1	71	
411.	Tuna, canned, oil pack, drained	3 oz.	85	167	25.0	7	1.7	60	0
412.	Tuna, canned, water pack, solids and liquid	3½ oz.	99	126	27.7	1	0.0	55	0
413.	Turkey, roast (light and dark mixed)	3 oz.	85	162	27.0	5	1.5	73	0
414.	Turnip, cooked, drained	1/2 c cubed	78	18	0.6	0	0.0	0	4
415.	Turnip greens, cooked drained	1/2 c	73	19	2.1	0	0.0	0	3
416.	Veal, cooked loin	3 oz.	85	199	22.0	11	4.0	90	0
417.	Veal cutlet, braised, broiled	3 oz.	85	185	23.0	9	4.0	109	0
418.	Vegetables, mixed, cooked	1 c	182	116	5.8	0	0.0	0	24
419.	Waffles	1 waffle	75	205	6.9	8	2.7	59	27
420.	Watermelon	1 c diced	160	42	0.8	0	0.0	0	10
421.	Wheat germ, plain toasted	1 tbsp	6	23	1.8	1	0.0	0	3
422.	Whiskey, gin, rum, vodka 90 proof	1/2 11 oz (jigger)	42	110	0	0	0.0	0	0
423.	Whopper, Burger King	1 sandwich	270	614	27.0	36	12.0	90	45
424.	Whopper with cheese, Burger King	1 sandwich	294	706	32.0	44	16.0	115	47
425.	Whopper, double, Burger King	1 sandwich	351	844	46.0	53	19.0	169	45
426.	Wine, dry table 12% alc.	3½ fl. oz.	102	87	0.1	0	0.0	0	4
427.	Wine, red dry 18.8% alc.	2 fl. oz.	59	81	0.1	0	0.0	0	5
428.	Yeast, brewers	1 tbsp	8	23	3.1	0	0.0	0	3
429.	Yogurt, fruit	1 c	227	231	9.9	2	1.6	10	43
430.	Yogurt, plain low fat	1 8-oz. container	226	113	7.7	4	2.3	15	12

"0" represents both less than 1 and 0

Sources:

Nutritive Value of American Foods in Common Units. Agriculture Handbook No. 456. U.S. Dept. of Agriculture. Washington, D.C. 1988.

Young, E. A., E. H. Brennan, and C. L. Irving, Guest Eds. Perspectives on Fast Foods. Public Health Currents, 19(1), 1979, Published by Ross Laboratories, Columbus, OH.

Dennison, D. The Dine System: the Nutrition Plan For Better Health. C. V. Mosby Company St. Louis, Missouri, 1982.

Pennington, S. A. T. and H. N. Church. Food Values of Portions Commonly Used. Harper and Row Publishers, New York, 1985.

Kullman, D. A. ABC Milligram Cholesterol Diet Guide. Merit Publications, Inc. North Miami Beach, Florida 1978.

Food Processor nutrient analysis software by Esha Corporation, P.O. Box 13028, Salem, Oregon, 97309. With permission.

Healthstyle:
A Self-Test*

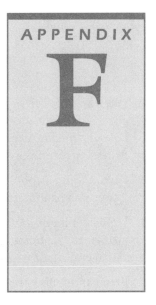

All of us want good health. But many of us do not know how to be as healthy as possible. Health experts now describe *lifestyle* as one of the most important factors affecting health. In fact, it is estimated that as many as seven of the ten leading causes of death could be reduced through common-sense changes in lifestyle. That's what this brief test, developed by the Public Health Service, is all about. Its purpose is simply to tell you how well you are doing to stay healthy. The behaviors covered in the test are recommended for most Americans. Some of them may not apply to persons with certain chronic diseases or handicaps, or to pregnant women. Such persons may require special instructions from their physicians.

Cigarette Smoking

If you *never smoke*, enter a score of 10 for this section and go to the next section on *Alcohol and Drugs*.

	Almost Always	Sometimes	Almost Never
1. I avoid smoking cigarettes.	2	1	0
2. I smoke only low tar and nicotine cigarettes *or* I smoke a pipe or cigars.	2	1	0

Smoking Score: _____

*Source: National Health Information Clearinghouse. Washington, D.C.

	Almost Always	Sometimes	Almost Never

Alcohol and Drugs

	Almost Always	Sometimes	Almost Never
1. I avoid drinking alcoholic beverages *or* I drink no more than 1 or 2 drinks a day.	2	1	0
2. I avoid using alcohol or other drugs (especially illegal drugs) as a way of handling stressful situations or the problems in my life.	2	1	0
3. I am careful not to drink alcohol when taking certain medicines (for example, medicine for sleeping, pain, colds, and allergies), or when pregnant.	2	1	0
4. I read and follow the label directions when using prescribed and over-the-counter drugs.	2	1	0

Alcohol and Drugs Score: _____

Eating Habits

	Almost Always	Sometimes	Almost Never
1. I eat a variety of foods each day, such as fruits and vegetables, whole grain breads and cereals, lean meats, dairy products, dry peas and beans, and nuts and seeds.	2	1	0
2. I limit the amount of fat, saturated fat, and cholesterol I eat (including fat on meats, eggs, butter, cream, shortenings, and organ meats such as liver).	2	1	0
3. I limit the amount of salt I eat by cooking with only small amounts, not adding salt at the table, and avoiding salty snacks.	2	1	0
4. I avoid eating too much sugar (especially frequent snacks of sticky candy or soft drinks).	2	1	0

Eating Habits Score: _____

Exercise/Fitness

	Almost Always	Sometimes	Almost Never
1. I maintain a desired weight, avoiding overweight and underweight.	2	1	0
2. I do vigorous exercises for 20–30 minutes at least 3 times a week (examples include running, swimming, brisk walking).	2	1	0
3. I do exercises that enhance my muscle tone for 15–30 minutes at least 3 times a week (examples include yoga and calisthenics).	2	1	0
4. I use part of my leisure time participating in individual, family, or team activities that increase my level of fitness (such as gardening, bowling, golf, and baseball).	2	1	0

Exercise/Fitness Score: _____

Stress Control

	Almost Always	Sometimes	Almost Never
1. I have a job or do other work that I enjoy.	2	1	0
2. I find it easy to relax and express my feelings freely.	2	1	0
3. I recognize early, and prepare for, events or situations likely to be stressful for me.	2	1	0
4. I have close friends, relatives, or others whom I can talk to about personal matters and call on for help when needed.	2	1	0
5. I participate in group activities (such as church and community organizations) or hobbies that I enjoy.	2	1	0

Stress Control Score: _____

Safety

		Almost Always	Sometimes	Almost Never
1.	I wear a seat belt while riding in a car.	2	1	0
2.	I avoid driving while under the influence of alcohol and other drugs.	2	1	0
3.	I obey traffic rules and the speed limit when driving.	2	1	0
4.	I am careful when using potentially harmful products or substances (such as household cleaners, poisons, and electrical devices).	2	1	0
5.	I avoid smoking in bed.	2	1	0

Safety Score: _____

What Your Scores Mean to YOU

Scores of 9 and 10 Excellent! Your answers show that you are aware of the importance of this area to your health. More important, you are putting your knowledge to work for you by practicing good health habits. As long as you continue to do so, this area should not pose a serious health risk. It's likely that you are setting an example for your family and friends to follow. Since you got a very high test score on this part of the test, you may want to consider other areas where your scores indicate room for improvement.

Scores of 6 to 8 Your health practices in this area are good, but there is room for improvement. Look again at the items you answered with a "Sometimes" or "Almost Never." What changes can you make to improve your score? Even a small change can often help you achieve better health.

Scores of 3 to 5 Your health risks are showing! Would you like more information about the risks you are facing and about why it is important for you to change these behaviors? Perhaps you need help in deciding how to successfully make the changes you desire. In either case, help is available.

Scores of 0 to 2 Obviously, you were concerned enough about your health to take the test, but your answers show that you may be taking serious and unnecessary risks with your health. Perhaps you are not aware of the risks and what to do about them. You can easily get the information and help you need to improve, if you wish. The next step is up to you.

YOU Can Start Right Now!

In the test you just completed were numerous suggestions to help you reduce your risk of disease and premature death. Here are some of the most significant:

Avoid cigarettes. Cigarette smoking is the single most important preventable cause of illness and early death. It is especially risky for pregnant women and their unborn babies. Persons who stop smoking reduce their risk of getting heart disease and cancer. So if you're a cigarette smoker, think twice about lighting that next cigarette. If you choose to continue smoking, try decreasing the number of cigarettes you smoke and switching to a low tar and nicotine brand.

Follow sensible drinking habits. Alcohol produces changes in mood and behavior. Most people who drink are able to control their intake of alcohol and to avoid undesired, and often harmful, effects. Heavy, regular use of alcohol can lead to cirrhosis of the liver, a leading cause of death. Also, statistics clearly show that mixing drinking and driving is often the cause of fatal or crippling accidents. So if you drink, do it wisely and in moderation. ***Use care in taking drugs.*** Today's greater use of drugs — both legal and illegal — is one of our most serious health risks. Even some drugs prescribed by your doctor can be dangerous if taken when drinking alcohol or before driving. Excessive or continued use of tranquilizers (or "pep pills") can cause physical and mental problems. Using or experimenting with illicit drugs such as marijuana, heroin, cocaine, and PCP may lead to a number of damaging effects or even death.

Eat sensibly. Overweight individuals are at greater risk for diabetes, gall bladder disease, and high blood pressure. So it makes good sense to maintain proper weight. But good eating habits also mean holding down the amount of fat (especially saturated fat), cholesterol, sugar and salt in your diet. If you must snack, try nibbling on fresh fruits and vegetables. You'll feel better — and look better, too.

Exercise regularly. Almost everyone can benefit from exercise — and there's some form of exercise almost everyone can do. (If you have any doubt, check first with your doctor.) Usually, as little as 20–30 minutes of vigorous exercise three times a week will help you have a healthier heart, eliminate excess weight, tone up sagging muscles, and sleep better. Think how much difference all these improvements could make in the way you feel!

Learn to handle stress. Stress is a normal part of living; everyone faces it to some degree. The causes of stress can be good or bad, desirable or undesirable (such as a promotion on the job or the loss of a spouse). Properly handled, stress need not be a problem. But unhealthy responses to stress — such as driving too fast or erratically, drinking too much, or prolonged anger or grief — can cause a variety of physical and mental problems. Even on a very busy day, find a few minutes to slow down and relax. Talking over a problem with someone you trust can often help you find a satisfactory solution. Learn to distinguish between things that are "worth fighting about" and things less important.

Be safety conscious. Think "safety first" at home, at work, at school, at play, and on the highway. Buckle seat belts and obey traffic rules. Keep poisons and weapons out of the reach of children, and keep emergency numbers by your telephone. When the unexpected happens, you'll be prepared.

Where Do You Go From Here:

Start by asking yourself a few frank questions: *Am I really doing all I can to be as healthy as possible? What steps can I take to feel better? Am I willing to begin now?* If you scored low in one or more *sections* of the test, decide what changes you want to make for improvement. You might pick that aspect of your lifestyle where you feel you have the best chance for success and tackle that one first. Once you have improved your score there, go on to other areas.

If you already have tried to change your health habits (to stop smoking or exercise regularly, for example), don't be discouraged if you haven't yet succeeded. The difficulty you have encountered may be due to influences you've never really thought about — such as advertising — or to a lack of support and encouragement. Understanding these influences is an important step toward changing the way they affect you.

There's Help Available. In addition to personal actions you can take on your own, there are community programs and groups (such as the YMCA or the local chapter of the American Heart Association) that can assist you and your family to make the changes you want to make. If you want to know more about these groups or about health risks, contact your local health department or the National Health Information Clearinghouse. There's a lot you can do to stay healthy or to improve your health — and there are organizations that can help you. Start a new HEALTHSTYLE today!

Bibliography

Allsen, P. E., J. M. Harrison and B. Vance. *Fitness for Life: An Individualized Approach.* Dubuque, IA: Wm. C. Brown, 1993.

Allsen, P. E. *Strength Training: Beginners, Bodybuilders, and Athletes.* Glenview, Illinois: Scott, Foresman and Company, 1987.

American College of Sports Medicine. *Guidelines for Exercise Testing and Prescription.* Philadelphia: Lea and Febiger, 1990.

American Heart Association. *1992 Heart and Stroke Facts.* Dallas, TX: The Association, 1992.

American College of Sports Medicine. "The Recommended Quantity and Quality of Exercise for Developing and Maintaining Cardiorespiratory and Muscular Fitness in Healthy Adults." *Medicine and Science in Sports and Exercise* 22:265–274, 1990.

American Cancer Society. *1992 Cancer Facts and Figures.* New York: The Society, 1992.

Arnheim, D. D. *Modern Principles of Athletic Training.* St. Louis, MO: Times Mirror/Mosby College Publishing, 1988.

Barnard, R. J. "Effects of Life-style Modification on Serum Lipids." *Archives of Internal Medicine* 151: 1389–1394, 1991.

Blair, S. N. *Living With Exercise.* Dallas: American Health Publishing Co., 1991.

Blair, S. N., H. W. Kohl III, R. S. Paffenbarger, Jr, D. G. Clark, K. H. Cooper, and L. W. Gibbons. "Physical Fitness and All-Cause Mortality: A Prospective Study of Healthy Men and Women." *Journal of the American Medical Association* 262:2395–2401, 1989.

Bouchard, C., and F. E. Johnson (Editors). *Fat Distribution During Growth and Later Health Outcomes.* New York: Alan R. Liss, 1988.

Brownell, K., and J. P. Forey. *Handbook of Eating Disorders.* New York: Basic Books, Inc., 1986.

Clark, B., W. Osness, W. W. K. Hoeger, M. Adrian, D. Raab, & R. Wiswell. Tests for fitness in older adults: AAHPERD fitness task force. *Journal of Physical Education, Recreation, and Dance* 60(3):66–71, 1989.

Cooper, K. H. "A Means of Assessing Maximal Oxygen Intake." *Journal of the American Medical Association* 203:201–204, 1968.

Cooper, K. H. *The Aerobics Program for Total Well-Being.* New York: Mount Evans and Co., 1982.

Cristian, J. L., and J. L. Greger. *Nutrition for Living.* Menlo Park, CA: The Benjamin/Cummings Publishing Co., 1991.

Drinkwater, B. L., B. Bruemner, and C. H. III Chestnut. "Menstrual History as a Determinant of Current Bone Density in Young Athletes." *Journal of the American Medical Association* 263:545–548, 1990.

Drinkwater, B. L. "Nutrition, Exercise, and Bone Health." Seattle, WA: Pacific Medical Center, 1990.

Helmrich, S. P., D. R. Ragland, R. W. Leung, and R. S. Paffenbarger. "Physical Activity and Reduced Occurrences of Non-Insulin-Dependent Diabetes Mellitus." *The New England Journal of Medicine* 325:147–152, 1991.

Hesson, J. L. *Weight Training for Life.* Englewood, Colorado: Morton Publishing Company, 1991.

Hoeger, W. W. K. *Lifetime Physical Fitness & Wellness: A Personalized Program.* Englewood, CO: Morton Publishing Company, 1992.

Hoeger, W. W. K. *Principles and Laboratories for Physical Fitness & Wellness.* Englewood, CO: Morton Publishing Company, 1991.

Hoeger, W. W. K. and D. R. Hopkins. A comparison between the sit and reach and the modified sit and reach in the measurement of flexibility in women. *Research Quarterly for Exercise & Sport* 63(2), 191–195, 1992.

Hopkins, D. R., and W. W. K. Hoeger. A comparison between the sit and reach and the modified sit and reach in the measurement of flexibility for males. *Journal of Applied Sport Science Research* 6(1), 7–10, 1992.

Jackson, A. S., and M. L. Pollock. "Generalized Equations for Predicting Body Density of Men." *British Journal of Nutrition* 40:497–504, 1978.

Jackson, A. S., M. L. Pollock, and A. Ward. "Generalized Equations for Predicting Body Density of Women." *Medicine and Science in Sports and Exercise* 3:175–182, 1980.

Karvonen, M. J., E Kentala, and O. Mustala. "The Effects of Training on the Heart Rate, a Longitudinal Study." *Annales Medicinae Experimetalis et Biologiae Fenniae* 35:307–315, 1957.

Kash, F. W., J. L. Boyer, S. P. Van Camp, L. S. Verity, and J. P. Wallace. "The Effect of Physical Activity on Aerobic Power in Older Men (A Longitudinal Study)." *The Physician and Sports Medicine* 18(4): 73–83, 1990.

Kline, G. et al. "Estimation of VO_{2max} from a one-mile track walk, gender, age, and body weight." *Medicine and Science in Sports and Exercise* 19(3):253–259, 1987.

Morgan, B. L. G., and R. Morgan. *Nutrition Tips.* Longmeadow Press, 1992.

National Academy of Sciences. "Diet and Health: Implications for Reducing Chronic Disease Risk." Washington, D. C. National Academy Press, 1989.

National Academy of Sciences. "Diet and Health: Implications for Reducing Chronic Disease Risk." Washington, D. C. National Academy Press, 1989.

Paffenbarger, R. S., R. T. Hyde, A. L. Wing, and C. H. Steinmetz. "A Natural History of Athleticism and Cardiovascular Health." *Journal of the American Medical Association* 252:491–495, 1984.

Remington, D., A. G. Fisher, and E. A. Parent. *How to Lower Your Fat Thermostat.* Provo, UT: Vitality House International, Inc. 1983.

Teitz, C. C. "Overuse Injuries," in *Scientific Foundations of Sports Medicine* (C. C. Teitz Editor, pp. 299–328). Philadelphia: B. C. Deckerm, 1989.

The Fallacies of Taking Supplementation. *Tufts University Diet & Nutrition Letter.* July 1987.

Thornton, J. S. "Feast or Famine: Eating Disorders in Athletes." *The Physician and Sportsmedicine* 18(4): 116–122, 1990.

Whitney, E. N. and E. M. N. Hamilton. *Understanding Nutrition.* St. Paul, MN: West Publishing Co., 1990.

Wiley, J. A. and T. C. Camacho. "Lifestyle and Future Health: Evidence from the Alameda County Study." *Preventive Medicine* 9:1–21, 1980.

Wilmore, J. H., and D. L. Costill. *Training for Sport and Activity.* Brown and Benchmark, 1988.

Your Back and How to Care For It. Kenilworth, NJ: Schering Corporation, 1965.

Glossary

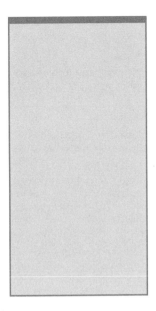

Acquired immunodeficiency syndrome (AIDS) Virus (HIV) that destroys the immune system.

Adipose tissue Fat cells.

Aerobic exercise Continuous exercise that involves major muscle groups and requires oxygen to produce the necessary energy (ATP) to carry out the activity.

Aerobic fitness *See* cardiovascular endurance.

AIDS *See* acquired immunodeficiency syndrome.

Alcohol (drinking alcohol) Known as ethyl alcohol, a depressant drug that affects the brain and slows down central nervous system activity.

Alcoholism Disease in which an individual loses control over drinking alcoholic-containing beverages.

Amenorrhea Cessation of regular menstrual flow.

Anaerobic exercise Exercise which does not require oxygen to produce the necessary energy (ATP) to carry out the activity.

Anorexia nervosa An eating disorder characterized by self-imposed starvation to lose and maintain very low body weight.

Antioxidants Compounds such as the vitamins C, E, beta-carotene (a precursor to vitamin A) and the mineral selenium which prevent oxygen from combining with other substances to which it may cause damage. Antioxidants are thought to play a key role in the prevention of heart disease and cancer.

Arteries Major vessels that carry blood away from the heart to bodily tissues.

Arteriosclerosis Hardening of the arteries.

Atherosclerosis Type of arteriosclerosis characterized by plaque formation or the buildup of fatty tissue in the inner layers of the wall of the arteries.

Atrophy A decrease in the size of a cell.

Ballistic or dynamic stretching (flexibility) Stretching exercises that are performed using jerky, rapid, and bouncy movements.

Basal metabolic rate The lowest level of oxygen consumption (uptake) necessary to sustain life.

Behavior modification A process to permanently change destructive or negative behaviors for positive behaviors that will lead to better health and well-being.

Benign Noncancerous.

Beta-carotene A precursor to vitamin A.

Blood pressure The pressure of the blood exerted against the walls of the arteries.

BMI See body mass index.

Body composition Term used in reference to the fat and nonfat components of the human body. Body composition is important in the assessment of recommended or "ideal" body weight.

Body density The weight of the body per unit volume.

Breathing techniques for relaxation Stress management technique where the individual concentrates on "breathing away" the tension and inhaling fresh air to the entire body.

Bulimia An eating disorder characterized by a pattern of binge eating and purging to attempt to lose and maintain low body weight.

CAD Coronary artery disease, see coronary heart disease.

Caffeine A central nervous system stimulating drug most frequently found in coffee, tea, and colas.

Calorie A unit to measure heat energy. A calorie (also referred to as small calorie) is the amount of heat necessary to raise the temperature of one gram of water one degree Centigrade. Short term for kilocalorie and it is used to measure the energy value of food and cost of physical activity.

Cancer Group of diseases characterized by uncontrolled growth and spread of abnormal cells into malignant tumors.

Capillary Smallest blood vessels carrying oxygenated blood in the body.

Carbohydrates Compounds containing carbon, hydrogen, and oxygen. Carbohydrates are the major source of energy for the human body.

Carcinogens Substances that contribute to the formation of cancers.

Cardiovascular diseases Diseases that affects the heart and the circulatory system (blood vessels). Examples of cardiovascular diseases are coronary heart disease, peripheral vascular disease, congenital heart disease, rheumatic heart disease, atherosclerosis, strokes, high blood pressure, and congestive heart failure.

Cardiovascular endurance The ability of the lungs, heart, and blood vessels to deliver adequate amounts of oxygen to the cells to meet the demands of prolonged (aerobic) physical activity.

Cardiovascular fitness *See* cardiovascular endurance.

Cardiovascular training zone Recommended exercise heart rate range to cause cardiovascular endurance development.

Cellulite Term frequently used in reference to fat deposits that "bulge out." These deposits are nothing but enlarged fat cells due to excessive accumulation of body fat.

CHD *See* coronary heart disease.

Chlamydia A sexually transmitted disease caused by a bacterial infection that can cause significant damage to the reproductive system and may occur without symptoms.

Cholesterol A waxy substance that is technically a steroid alcohol found only in animal fats and oil.

Chronic diseases Diseases that develop over a prolonged period of time, usually associated to unhealthy lifestyle factors (hypertension, atherosclerosis, coronary disease, strokes, diabetes, and cancer).

Chronic obstructive pulmonary disease (COPD) An air flow limiting disease that includes diseases such as chronic bronchitis and emphysema.

Chronological age Actual age of the individual (*also see* functional age).

Cocaine 2-beta-carbomethoxy-3-betabenozoxytropane — the primary psychoactive ingredient derived from coca plant leaves. Also referred to as coke, C, snow, blow, toot, flake, Peruvian lady, white girl, and happy dust.

Coenzyme Nonprotein molecule required in enzyme reactions.

Complex carbohydrates Carbohydrates formed by three or more simple sugar molecules linked together, also referred to as polysaccharides. Commonly used to designate foods high in starch.

Concentric muscle contraction Shortening of fibers during muscle contraction.

Congenital heart disease Heart defects present at birth.

Coronary arteries Arteries that supply the myocardium or heart muscle with oxygen and nutrients.

Coronary heart disease Disease caused by the obstruction of the coronary arteries by plaque formation (also see atherosclerosis).

Cruciferous vegetables Plants that produce cross-shaped leaves (cauliflower, broccoli, cabbage, Brussels sprouts, and kohlrabi). These vegetables seem to have a protective effect against cancer.

Dehydration A loss of body water below normal volume.

Deoxyribonucleic acid (DNA) Genetic material, substance of which genes are made.

Diabetes mellitus Condition where the blood glucose is unable to enter the cells because the pancreas either totally stops producing insulin or produces an insufficient amount for the body's needs.

Diastolic blood pressure Pressure exerted by the blood against the walls of the arteries during the relaxation phase (diastole) of the heart.

Dietary fiber Fiber in plant foods that cannot be digested by the human body.

DNA *See* deoxyribonucleic acid.

Dysmenorrhea Painful menstruation.

Eccentric muscle contraction Lengthening of fibers during muscle contraction.

ECG   *See* electrocardiogram.

EKG   *See* electrocardiogram.

Elastic elongation (flexibility)   Refers to an elastic or temporary lengthening of soft tissue (muscles, tendons, and ligaments).

Electrocardiogram (ECG or EKG)   A recording of the electrical activity of the heart.

Emphysema   Pulmonary disease caused by distention (overinflation) of the alveoli.

Endorphines   Morphine-like substances released from the pituitary gland in the brain during prolonged aerobic exercise. They are thought to induce feelings of euphoria and natural well-being.

Endurance   *See* cardiovascular endurance and muscular endurance.

Enzyme   A catalyst that facilitates chemical reactions.

Epidemiology   Science that studies the relationship between diverse factors (lifestyle and environmental) and the occurrence of disease.

Essential fat   Minimal amount of body fat needed for normal physiological functions. It constitutes about 3 percent of the total fat in men and 12 percent in women.

Estrogen   Female sex hormone. Essential for bone formation and bone density conservation.

Eumenorrhea   Normal menstrual cycle.

Exercise adherence   Initiating and participating in an exercise program for life.

Exercise electrocardiogram   An exercise test during which the workload is gradually increased (until the subject reaches maximal fatigue) with blood pressure and twelve-lead electrocardiographic monitoring throughout the test.

Exercise intolerance   Exercise conducted at intensity levels well beyond a person's functional capacity leading to symptoms such as very rapid or irregular heart rate, labored breathing, nausea, vomiting, lightheadedness, headaches, dizziness, pale skin, flushness, excessive weakness, lack of energy, shakiness, sore muscles, cramps, and tightness in the chest.

Exercise readiness   A person's level of preparedness to initiate and adhere to an exercise program.

Exercise tolerance test   *See* exercise electrocardiogram.

Fats   Compounds made by a combination of triglycerides.

Fiber   A form of complex carbohydrate made up of plant material that cannot be digested by the human body.

Fight or flight mechanism   Physiological response of the body to stress which prepares the individual to take action by stimulating the vital defense systems.

Flexibility   The ability of a joint to move freely through its full range of motion.

Free fatty acids (FFA)   Fatty acids released by the breakdown of triglycerides.

Free radicals   *See* oxygen free radicals.

Functional age   Physiological age of the individual. Usually lower than the chronological (actual) age in fit people and vice versa in unfit people.

Genetics   Science that studies genetic or hereditary conditions.

Genital warts   A sexually transmitted disease caused by a viral infection. Genital warts increase the risk of cervical cancer. Enlargement and spread of the warts leads to obstruction of the urethra, vagina, and anus.

Glucose   Blood sugar, type of carbohydrate (monosaccharide), a primary source of energy for the human body.

Glucose intolerance   Inability to properly metabolize glucose.

Glycogen   Form of carbohydrate (polysaccharide) storage in muscle.

Gonorrhea   A sexually transmitted disease caused by a bacterial infection that can lead to pelvic inflammation in women, infertility, widespread bacterial infection, heart damage, arthritis in men and women, and blindness in children born to infected women.

HDL   *See* high density lipoprotein.

Health-fitness standards   Minimum fitness standards to significantly decrease the risk of disease.

Health promotion   Programs aimed at helping people develop healthy lifestyle behaviors that will lead to a higher state of wellness.

Health-related fitness   Refers to fitness components that when enhanced lead to better health (cardiovascular endurance, body composition, muscular strength and endurance, and muscular flexibility).

Heart attack   *See* myocardial infarct

Heart rate reserve   The difference between the maximal heart rate and the resting heart rate.

Heat cramps   Muscle cramps caused by heat-induced changes in electrolyte balance in muscle cells.

Heat exhaustion   Heat-related condition; symptoms include fainting, dizziness, profuse sweating, cold clammy skin, headaches and a rapid, weak pulse.

Heat stroke   Heat-related emergency; symptoms include serious disorientation, warm dry skin, no sweating, rapid full pulse, vomiting, diarrhea, unconsciousness, and high body temperature.

Hemoglobin Protein-iron compound in red blood cells that transports oxygen in the blood.

Herpes A sexually transmitted disease caused by a viral infection (herpes simplex virus types I and II). No known cure is available for the disease. The disease is characterized by the appearance of sores on the mouth, genitals, rectum, or other parts of the body.

High density lipoprotein (HDL) Cholesterol-transporting molecules in the blood. High HDL-cholesterol (good cholesterol) seems to offer protection against some forms of cardiovascular disease.

HIV *See* human immunodeficiency virus.

Human immunodeficiency virus (HIV) Virus that causes acquired immunodeficiency syndrome (AIDS).

Hydrostatic weighing Underwater weighing technique to assess body composition, including percent body fat.

Hyperlipidemia Elevated blood fats or lipids.

Hypertension Chronically elevated blood pressure.

Hypertrophy An increase in the size of the cell (for example, muscle hypertrophy).

Hypokinetic disease Diseases associated with a lack of physical activity (hypertension, coronary heart disease, obesity, and diabetes).

Insulin Hormone secreted by the pancreas that increases the absorption and utilization of glucose by the body.

Isokinetic contraction Muscular contraction at a constant velocity.

Isokinetic training Strength-training method where the speed of the muscle contraction is kept constant because the equipment (machine) provides an accommodating resistance to match the user's force (maximal) through the range of motion.

Isometric training Strength-training method that refers to a muscle contraction producing little or no movement, such as pushing or pulling against immovable objects.

Isotonic training Strength-training method that refers to a muscle contraction with movement, such as lifting an object over the head.

Kilocalorie A unit to measure heat energy. A kilocalorie (kcal) or large calorie is the amount of heat necessary to raise the temperature of one kilogram of water one degree Centigrade. One kcal equals 1,000 calories.

LDL *See* low density lipoprotein.

Lean body mass Body weight without body fat.

Low density lipoprotein (LDL) Cholesterol-transporting molecules in the blood. High LDL-cholesterol (bad cholesterol) seems to increase the risk for some forms of cardiovascular disease.

Malignant melanoma Deadliest of all types of skin cancer. Tumors grow at a rapid rate and readily spread to other parts of the body if not treated at an early stage.

Marijuana A psychoactive drug prepared from a mixture of crushed leaves, flowers, small branches, stems, and seeds from the hemp plant cannabis sativa. Also referred to as pot and grass.

Maximal oxygen uptake (Max VO$_{2max}$) The maximal amount of oxygen that the body is able to utilize per minute of physical activity, commonly expressed in ml/kg/min. The best indicator of cardiovascular or aerobic fitness.

Meditation Stress management technique used to gain control over one's attention, clearing the mind and blocking out the stressor(s) responsible for the increased tension.

Melanoma A malignant tumor.

METS (metabolic equivalents) A measurement unit of resting energy expenditure. One MET is the equivalent of 3.5 ml/kg/min.

Metabolism All energy and material transformations that occur within living cells necessary to sustain life.

Minerals Inorganic elements found in the body and in food which are essential for normal body functions.

Mitochondria Structures within the cells where energy transformations take place.

Monounsaturated fat Fatty acids with only one double bond found along the carbon atom chain.

Motor skill-related fitness Refers to fitness components that when improved lead to enhanced athletic performance (agility, balance, coordination, power, reaction time, and speed).

Muscle fiber A muscle cell.

Muscular endurance (localized muscular endurance) The ability of a muscle to exert submaximal force repeatedly over a period of time (for example, 30 repetitions on a bench press exercise). It usually implies a specific muscle group (chest, thighs, abdominals).

Muscular flexibility *See* flexibility.

Muscular strength The ability of a muscle to exert maximum force against resistance (for example, 1 repetition maximum or 1 RM on the bench press exercise).

Myocardial infarct Death of part of the myocardium.

Myocardium Heart muscle.

Nicotine Poisonous compound found in tobacco leaves.

Nonmelanoma Nonmalignant tumor.

Nutrient Substance found in food that provide energy, regulate metabolism, and help with growth and repair of body tissues.

Nutrient density Ratio of nutrients to calories in food.

Nutrition Science that studies the relationship of foods to optimal health and performance.

Obesity Refers to an excessive accumulation of body fat, usually about 30 percent above recommended body weight according to body size.

Oligomenorrhea Irregular menstrual cycles.

Omega-3 fatty acids Polyunsaturated fatty acids found primarily in cold water seafood and are thought to be effective in lowering blood cholesterol and triglycerides.

One repetition maximum (1 RM) The maximal amount of resistance (weight) that an individual is able to lift in a single effort.

Osteoporosis Softening, deterioration, or loss of total body bone.

Overload principle Key training concept which states that the demands placed on a system (cardiovascular, muscular) must be systematically and progressively increased over a period of time to cause physiologic adaptation (development or improvement).

Oxygen free radicals Substances formed during metabolism which attack and damage proteins and lipids, in particular the cell membrane and DNA; leading to the development of diseases such as heart disease, cancer, and emphysema. Antioxidants are believed to exert a protective effect by absorbing free radicals before they can cause damage and also by interrupting the sequence of reactions once damage has begun.

Percent body fat Term used in body composition assessment. It represents the total amount of fat in the body based on the person's weight. It includes both essential and storage fat.

Physical fitness (health-related) The general capacity to adapt and respond favorably to physical effort, implying that individuals are physically fit when they can meet the ordinary as well as the unusual demands of daily life safely and effectively without being overly fatigued, and still have energy left for leisure and recreational activities.

Physical-fitness standards Required standards to achieve a high level of fitness.

Plastic elongation (flexibility) Refers to a permanent lengthening of soft tissue (capsules, tendons, and ligaments).

PNF *See* proprioceptive neuromuscular facilitation.

Polyunsaturated fat Fatty acids with two or more double bonds along the carbon atom chain.

Proprioceptive neuromuscular facilitation (PNF — for flexibility development) Stretching technique where muscles are progressively stretched out with intermittent isometric contractions.

Protein Complex organic compounds containing nitrogen and formed by combinations of amino acids. Proteins are the main substances used in the body to build and repair tissues such as muscles, blood, internal organs, skin, hair, nails, and bones. They are also part of hormones, antibodies, and enzymes.

RDA *See* recommended dietary allowances.

Recommended dietary allowances (RDA) Daily recommended intakes of nutrients for normal, healthy people in the United States.

Repetition (in strength training) The number of times that a given resistance is performed (for example, 12 repetitions on the bench press exercise).

Repetition maximum (in strength training) The maximum number of repetitions (RM) that can be performed with a specific resistance or weight (for example, 10 RM with 150 pounds).

Resistance (in strength training) The amount of weight that is lifted.

Resting metabolic rate Amount of energy (expressed in milliliters of oxygen per minute or total calories per day) required during resting conditions to sustain proper body function.

Risk factors Lifestyle and genetic factors that may lead to disease.

Saturated fat Fatty acids with carbon atoms fully saturated with hydrogens, therefore only single bonds link the carbon atoms on the chain. High intake of saturated fats increases the risk for coronary heart disease.

Serum cholesterol Blood cholesterol level.

Set (in strength training) A number of repetitions (1 set of 12 repetitions).

Sexually transmitted diseases (STDs) Diseases spread through sexual contact.

Shin Splints   Injury to the lower leg characterized by pain and irritation in the shin region or front of the leg.

Simple carbohydrates   Carbohydrates formed by simple or double sugar units with little nutritive value (for example, candy, pop, cakes, etc.), frequently denoted as sugars. Simple carbohydrates are divided into monosaccharides and disaccharides.

Skill-related fitness   Refers to additional fitness components that enhance athletic performance (agility, balance, coordination, reaction time, power, and speed).

Skinfold thickness   Technique to assess body composition, including percent body fat, by measuring the thickness of a double fold of skin at different body sites.

Slow-sustained or static stretching (flexibility)   Stretching technique where the muscles are gradually lengthened through a joint's complete range of motion and the final position is held for a few seconds.

Specificity of training   Training programs must be specifically aimed at the desired outcome. This is accomplished by training with the specific activity that the person is attempting to improve (aerobic, anaerobic, strength, flexibility).

Spiritual well-being   An affirmation of life in a relationship with God, self, community, and environment that nurtures and celebrates wholeness.

Spot reducing   Theory that claims that exercising a specific body part (for example, abdominal or midsection of the body) will result in significant fat reduction in that area. It does not work! (See Chapter 7 — Exercise: The Key to Successful Weight Loss and Weight Maintenance).

STDs   *See* sexually transmitted diseases

Storage fat   Body fat in excess of the essential fat. It is stored in adipose tissue.

Strength   *See* muscular strength.

Strength training   A conditioning program that requires the use of weights to help increase muscular strength, endurance, power, and/or body size.

Stress test   *See* exercise electrocardiogram.

Stress   The nonspecific response of the human organism to any demand that is placed upon it.

Stressor   Reaction of the organism to a stress-causing event.

Syphilis   A sexually transmitted disease caused by a bacterial infection. During the last stage of the disease, some people will suffer from paralysis, crippling, blindness, heart disease, brain damage, insanity, and even death.

Systolic blood pressure   Pressure exerted by the blood against the walls of the arteries during the forceful contraction (systole) of the heart.

Tar   Chemical compound that forms during the burning of tobacco leaves.

Testosterone   Male sex hormone.

Triglycerides   Fats formed by glycerol and three fatty acids.

U.S. RDA   The United States recommended daily allowances. Derived from the RDA and developed as a standard for nutrition labeling.

Vasoconstriction   Narrowing or clamping down of blood vessels.

Vasodilation   Widening or opening up of blood vessels.

Veins   Major vessels that carry blood back to the heart.

Very low density lipoprotein (VLDL)   Triglyceride, cholesterol and phospholipid-transporting molecules in the blood. Only a small amount of cholesterol is carried by the VLDL molecules.

Vitamins   Organic substances essential for normal metabolism, growth, and development of the body.

VLDL   *See* very low density lipoprotein.

VO$_{2max}$ *See* maximal oxygen uptake

Waist-to-Hip Ratio   Test designed by a panel of scientists appointed by the National Academy of Sciences and the Dietary Guidelines Advisory Council for the U.S. Departments of Agriculture and Health and Human Services to assess potential risk for diseases associated with obesity.

Weight training   A conditioning program that requires the use of weights to help increase muscular strength, endurance, power, and/or body size.

Wellness   The constant and deliberate effort to stay healthy and achieve the highest potential for well-being. Implies the adoption of healthy lifestyle factors that will decrease the risk for disease and enhance well-being.

Workload   A given level of exercise intensity or physical performance.

Yellow fat cells   Cells used for fat storage (stores of energy in the form of fat).

Index